Children with Social, Emotional and Behavioural Difficulties and Communication Problems

Children with Social, Emotional and Behavioural Difficulties and Communication Problems

There is Always a Reason

SECOND EDITION

Melanie Cross

Jessica Kingsley *Publishers*
London and Philadelphia

This edition published in 2011
by Jessica Kingsley Publishers
73 Collier Street
London N1 9BE, UK
and
400 Market Street, Suite 400
Philadelphia, PA 19106, USA

www.jkp.com

First edition published in 2004

Library of Congress Cataloging in Publication Data
Cross, Melanie.
Children with social, emotional and behavioural difficulties and communication
problems : there is always a reason / Melanie Cross. -- 2nd ed.
p. cm.
Includes bibliographical references and index.
ISBN 978-1-84905-129-3 (alk. paper)
1. Communicative disorders in children. 2. Children--Language. 3. Problem children--
Language. 4. Emotional problems of children. 5. Behavior disorders in children. I. Title.
RJ496.C67C766 2011
618.92'855--dc22
2011006807

British Library Cataloguing in Publication Data
A CIP catalogue record for this book is available from the British Library

ISBN 978 1 84905 129 3
eISBN 978 0 85700 326 3

This second edition is dedicated to my wonderful family, who have made me realise the true value of emotions and communication.

Acknowledgements

I owe a great debt of gratitude to all of those who have helped me learn everything new in this edition. That includes the adults, children and young people at the Integrated Services Programme (ISP). It has been a privilege to work with those who have helped in the development of the speech and language therapy service for children with social, emotional, behavioural and communication difficulties (SEBCD), and with those who have inspired me with their dedication to improving the circumstances of children who have had challenging lives.

I am also indebted to those I have worked with at I CAN. Our efforts to raise the profile of children with communication problems has led to opportunities to collaborate with and learn from many wonderful people and further research.

I am also lucky to work with SLT students and staff at City University who constantly make me think. They are enthusiastic in their efforts to find effective ways to work with those who have communication difficulties.

I'm grateful to many others who have helped in the process of writing this book, with ideas, proofreading and editing and, indeed, comments about the first edition. I am also grateful to those who have supported me in my training in video interaction guidance, a very useful approach for children with SEBCD.

Contents

Introduction

This is the second edition of the book I needed when I began to work with children and young people with social, emotional and behavioural difficulties (SEBD). As a speech and language therapist, I knew about communication, but I found it hard to understand how communication problems related to SEBD. Was there a link between the two and, if so, why? I had difficulty initially persuading other professionals that communication problems were significant for these young people; after all, many of them had had severely disrupted lives and little formal education, so did a few additional speech and language problems matter? The short answer, and the main thrust of this book, is that, yes, they do matter. Speech and language problems matter because emotional and language development are linked and intertwined. Communication problems can impair people's ability to interact, manage their behaviour, learn and think. Language and communication skills are central to us as human beings, and where there are communication problems, young people have great difficulty achieving their potential. Conversely, providing them with opportunities to learn communication skills can increase their access to education, improve their interactions and give them tools to think about emotions and to construct a narrative about themselves.

I felt a new edition was necessary, as there has been so much new research and thinking surrounding this work. The link between behaviour and communication is increasingly obvious to people, but there is still much to do. I still regularly meet children and young people with SEBD who have undetected and unaddressed communication problems.

My initial impressions of working with children with SEBD were mixed. I was horrified one morning by the sight of a nine-year-old having a violent 'temper tantrum' like a two-year-old. He was expressing rage beyond anything I had ever experienced, and he appeared to be totally out of control. Of course it wasn't really something that had happened in the playground which had caused this reaction but something grim in his past, but that wasn't immediately obvious. I was impressed by the adults with him who managed to gently 'sandwich' him between them on a bench until he was able to calm down. They could see beyond the appalling behaviour to the terrified child. They didn't want to punish him but help him understand that he was safe and that they didn't want him to get hurt. As I got to know this boy, I found out that he had communication problems which meant that although he was bright, he was not able to say what he wanted to very easily and he did not always understand what others said to him.

These communication problems had not been identified, even though they were often the cause of great frustration for him. This communication frustration was an additional load on a young man who was already struggling with coming to terms with his past, who was unable to make friends and who was not progressing in school.

More recently I worked with another boy who has very complex difficulties but who has been able to learn ways to start conversations and play with his peers without resorting to violence – small but important steps in the right direction.

Much of this book is about seeing beyond the behaviour. There is always a reason for the bad behaviour, and dealing with those reasons changes the behaviour. This book aims to enable anyone working with children and young people who have social, emotional and behavioural problems to be aware of potential communication difficulties, recognise some and have some understanding of how the struggling child could be responded to in a positive way.

There is evidence for a strong link between emotional development and language development. Since emotional and communication difficulties often coexist, Chapter 1 of this book begins with ideas about how the two typically develop and how they might be linked. The relative importance of factors within the child and within his or her environment is discussed. Although there are various theories of language development, the importance of interaction with the significant person who responds to the infant's expressions of his or her needs and feelings is key. The impetus to communicate may be innate, but children will not learn to interact verbally if no one is able to interact with them responsively.

Attachment theory describes how a reciprocal relationship with a significant adult is important for emotional development. Securely attached children use more complex language than maltreated children. Therefore, a sensitive and contingent relationship between child and carer seems to be important for both emotional and communication development. If children do not experience responsive interactions early on, much of their subsequent development is at risk.

Given that emotional and language development are probably linked, is it also the case that problems in one area can affect the other? Chapter 2 considers the co-occurrence of emotional and communication difficulties. It is likely that the relationship between these two is complex. Children and young people who have communication problems are at risk of social emotional, behavioural and psychiatric problems. Difficulties in language comprehension seem to be a high risk factor for the development of psychiatric problems.

There is less evidence that social, emotional and behavioural problems lead to communication difficulties, although selective mutism, where a young person is only able to communicate in some situations, might be an exception. Communication problems are also an integral part of some difficulties such as autism spectrum disorder. Attention deficit hyperactivity disorder (ADHD) is also very closely associated with communication problems. It may be that some kinds of communication difficulties and mental health difficulties, such as ADHD and Tourette's syndrome, are both due to executive function deficits; that is, limitations in skills of self-regulation, which include the development of 'private speech.'

In addition to these possible links there are also many factors which could lead to both SEBD and communication problems. Adverse environmental factors, such as perinatal complications, psychosocial stress and those accompanying low socio-economic status, can affect language and emotional development. Interaction and, in particular, attachment difficulties also seem to be implicated in atypical emotional and language development. The effects of child abuse are also devastating for both emotional and language development. Furthermore, learning difficulties can lead to both emotional and communication problems. For some children, many factors contribute to the difficult development of SEBD and communication problems. It is necessary to capture the complexity of these factors if we are to understand these young people and intervene effectively.

Although there are strong links between language and emotional development, evidence suggests that large numbers of children with social, emotional and behavioural problems have unidentified communication problems. It is also the case that children with SEBD are perhaps ten times more likely to experience communication problems than other children and young people. Chapter 3 considers the implications of this tendency.

The significance of such undetected communication difficulties is discussed in terms of its negative impact on behaviour, emotional development, educational progress and social interactions. The first effect of communication difficulties for a child or young person is an increase in anxiety and frustration, which can manifest itself in unacceptable behaviour. Communication problems have also been shown to have a devastating effect on the development of literacy skills, which can further increase frustration and lower self-esteem.

Children with previously undetected communication problems are at risk of being misunderstood, their inappropriate responses seen as a lack of compliance rather than a lack of understanding. Children and young people with undetected communication problems may be subjected to inappropriate, verbally based interventions. While children's communication problems remain undetected, their behaviour may be misinterpreted as lack of co-operation or defiance. It is possible that identifying and addressing communication problems in this population could reduce social, emotional and behavioural problems.

It is important to think about why communication problems are undetected in this population. It may be that those affected have more obvious difficulties with their behaviour. Parents of children with undetected communication problems may themselves be disadvantaged and therefore not in a good position to identify difficulties in their children. A further complication is that communication problems can change in nature over time, making them more difficult to identify.

The main reason communication difficulties remain undetected is that there is a general lack of awareness and training about such problems and their potential negative effects. Professionals who work with children and young people who have social, emotional and behavioural difficulties may not be looking for communication difficulties, and consequently don't find them. So a communication assessment should be a routine part of work with a child or young person who has SEBD, and any difficulties should be addressed, particularly as good communication skills are protective against mental health difficulties.

Chapter 4 concentrates on the reasons for the link between language and social disadvantage, and focuses on vulnerable groups such as children who have been abused and neglected, those in public care, children excluded from school, young offenders and those not in employment, education or training. Limited communication skills put these children and young people at further risk of social exclusion.

Chapter 5 considers the practical problems involved in the identification and assessment of communication problems. It is important to identify communication problems because of their negative and potentially long-term effects on thinking, learning and interaction; however, there is no consensus about how to do this. No two children or young people have the same communication problems, and any or all areas of communication can be affected. Therefore, a variety of assessments are necessary to gain a clear picture of a young person's strengths and needs.

Assessment is further complicated by the various definitions of communication problems. This chapter goes on to discuss the advantages and disadvantages of various types of assessment approaches.

The self-assessment by the child or young person as well as contributions by others who know them are very important, and ways of collecting this type of information are discussed. It is necessary to consider the ways in which children and young people with social, emotional and behavioural problems might respond to formal and informal assessment, and to be sensitive to them. Both lack of co-operation and eagerness to please could influence the results. It is crucial to consider how a young person with previously undetected communication problem might feel about assessment. Some are relieved because they knew there was 'something going on' but did not know what. Others feel that they are 'just stupid'; sensitive explanations of the nature of communication problems are necessary.

The most useful assessment is likely to come from a variety of approaches which lead to a holistic view of the child's or young persons' communication strengths and needs. There is evidence that even just the recognition of a communication problem can improve interactions because it can alter expectations; this is an example of how knowledge can promote understanding.

Chapter 6, 'What Can be Done', is practically based. It starts with ideas about what can be done by anyone working with children with social, emotional, behavioural and communication difficulties (SEBCD). Since positive, responsive interactions are crucial in the development of communication, emotion and, indeed, thinking skills, these sorts of interactions contribute to good outcomes for children with SEBCD.

Often children and young people behave in unacceptable ways because they have skills gaps. We can teach them skills to behave well as we would teach them anything else. This includes a focus on emotional-literacy skills, positive-thinking skills and, of course, communication skills such as narratives and social communication skills.

The last section concentrates on specific interventions, either for groups or individuals, often delivered by experts.

There is a need for far more research; however, much can be done given the current state of knowledge:

- Children and young people with social, emotional and behavioural difficulties should be screened for communication difficulties, which have negative effects on their social, emotional and educational development.

- Everyone working with children with SEBCD should know how to identify communication problems, modify their communication and the tasks they set and provide communication-friendly environments where children and young adults can develop their skills.

- Speech and language therapy should be available for children and young people with SEBCD.

- Collaborative working is vital to help young people with social, emotional, behavioural and communication difficulties to achieve their potential.

Chapter 1

Are Language and Emotional Development Linked?

Perhaps the most important message in this book is that young people who have social, emotional and behavioural problems are also very likely to have communication problems. More worryingly, these communication problems often go unrecognised (Cohen *et al.* 1998). It is also the case that young people who have difficulty learning language often develop social, emotional and behavioural difficulties. In order to understand this apparent link, we need to consider how emotional and language development usually occurs, and how thinking skills are related developmentally. An understanding of this relationship can also provide us with ideas about how we might help young people with social, emotional, behavioural and communication difficulties (SEBCD).

What are language and communication skills?

Before considering how language and communication develops, we need to think about the necessary component skills. Communication is a complex process, but we tend not to notice its intricacy: for most of us it just happens, rapidly and without conscious thought. Language is easy to take for granted because it is everywhere; we use language to talk about and organise our experiences, to build relationships, to learn about the world and ourselves, and to think, manage our emotions and imagine. There are of course many types of language: spoken, written, symbol-based and signed.

The skills necessary for communication can be divided into *form*, *content* and *use*. It is also necessary to be able to use these skills and understand when someone else uses them.

Form

The form of any communication system is basically its structure. To be an effective communicator, you need to be able to use and understand form effectively. In spoken language, form includes the way sounds are ordered to make intelligible words. If someone has difficulty with this, it may be described as a 'speech difficulty', 'articulation problem' or phonological disorder'. Some of the component skills necessary for this are detailed in Table 1.1.

Another part of form is the grammar of language. It is important to get the words in the right order if we are going to make sense; for example, 'Tony ate it' and 'It ate Tony' mean very different things. The sequence of sentences and ideas in a narrative is equally important. Grammar also includes word beginnings, as in moral/amoral, or endings, which can indicate the tense of words, such as, 'I walk' or 'I walked'; and plurals, for example 'I've got a cat' or 'I've got cats'. Grammar, in this sense, is not prescriptive; it is not about what someone has decided is the correct way to speak. Rather, it is about rules that help us understand each other. Someone's difficulty with form might be described as a 'language' difficulty.

Table 1.1 Form		
	Understanding	Expressive
Sound system	Being able to hear the difference between speech sounds and words which sound similar, e.g. conclusion and solution	Having clear, fluent speech
Grammar	Being able to recognise and understand the difference between sentences, e.g. 'You can have a sweet' and 'You can have sweets' and 'She hit him' and 'She was hit by him'	Using grammar appropriately, e.g. 'Yesterday I saw him' rather than 'Yesterday I sawed him'
Narrative	Understanding the sequence of events in a story or a set of instructions	Organising and expressing ideas in a logical or chronological order

Content

The content of communication is its meaning. A full knowledge of the structure of language is of little use unless you are also able to convey and understand meaning, which requires knowledge of vocabulary. We also share meaning through idiomatic and abstract phrases like 'Keep your hair on' and by implying meaning when we say, for example, 'This is a mess' and hope someone might clear it up. Some examples of the skills necessary to understand and use the content of language are in Table 1.2.

Table 1.2 Content		
	Understanding	Expressive
Conveying meaning	Being able to understand words, concepts and implied meanings. For example, when the PE teacher says, 'Hit it with a bat', it is unlikely that they mean use a small flying rodent Recognising that idioms such as 'Don't hit the ceiling' shouldn't be taken literally	Being able to find the words you need and using them appropriately in context

Use

Knowledge of the structure and content of language are important, but they are not enough. Successful communicators also need to be able to use language in a social context. These verbal and non-verbal communication skills begin to develop before spoken language and form the basis of our interactions. To be a successful communicator, you need to use eye contact and facial expression. You also need to be able to recognise the nuances of meaning that non-verbal communication provide, and let that influence your response. There are subtle, unwritten rules about how conversations work. Context guides how we communicate; for example, we would talk to a child in a museum very differently to the way that we would talk to our best friend in a pub.

Some of the component skills necessary to use language to communicate are detailed in Table 1.3.

Table 1.3 Use		
	Understanding	Expressive
Being able to use language to communicate appropriately in context	Listening and asking for clarification Understanding the speaker's point of view Knowing when it's appropriate to take a turn Looking at and understanding non-verbal feedback	Being able to give the right amount of relevant information Staying on topic Taking turns in a conversation 'Repairing' if communication breaks down Demonstrating understanding by giving verbal and non-verbal feedback Knowing what can be said to a peer and to a teacher Negotiating a part in a game or activity

In order to communicate well, you need:

- speech which is easily understood
- sentences which are constructed appropriately
- sentences joined logically to make a narrative or story
- memory skills to help you plan what you want to say
- to know and retrieve the appropriate vocabulary and abstract language
- to understand what others say
- interaction skills and an understanding of the rules of conversation.

And you have to be able to do all of these at once!

The interactive element must never be overlooked. Communication involves joint attention, joint interest and a desire to share understanding; it involves initiation and reciprocation (Griffiths 2002).

Language development

Learning to use language to communicate is an impressive achievement when you consider all the skills that have to be learned and used simultaneously. What is even more remarkable is that most children learn language very rapidly. The process seems to start before birth. Babies can hear the rhythms and language of their mother's speech before they are born and prefer these once they are born. Soon after birth, babies are more interested in people than anything else, and this includes what they say. Gradually through their first year, infants focus on speech that is directed at them, and they experiment with making sounds. Between 6 and 12 months of age, babies recognise the most common language in use around them and they focus on that, losing their ability to hear the difference between speech sounds in other languages. In fact, those who are better than other children at identifying the sounds of their own language are more likely to have more advanced language skills at three years of age (Kuhl *et al.* 2005). At ten months, babies babble using sounds from the language they hear most. Babies begin to understand words at eight to ten months of age; this is amazing, given the number of possible meanings for any particular word.

It takes longer for them to use words to express themselves. This gap between understanding and using language continues, as children tend to be able to understand more language than they are able to express. First words appear at around a year, and by two years old, toddlers are linking words (Bates, Thal and Janowsky 1992). At two, a toddler may be learning nine new words every day (this is described as 'fast-mapping' or the 'vocabulary spurt'); between two and three years of age, most grammatical features are learned, which is known as the 'grammatical explosion' (Fenson *et al.* 1994). At the same time, children are learning how to use language in interactions with other people. Even in these preschool years children can take turns in a conversation and keep on topic. By two, they can use different sorts of language to interact with their mothers and fathers.

Words for feelings and other mental states, such as what is wanted, thought or felt, are also learnt between the ages of two and three. Children first use these mental-state words to refer to themselves, but by the time they are three, they can usually use them to describe others.

As well as developing language rapidly, most children are able to be very creative with it. Children make up words if they don't know them; e.g. 'blow ball' for 'balloon'. Similarly, deaf children create signs if they don't know the ones they need. Small children may overextend the use of a word, which can cause amusement, for example when they call all men 'daddy'.

By about three years of age, children are able to construct simple narratives with clear structure which can help them reflect, solve problems and consider future events.

Most children starting school can understand 10,000 to 20,000 words, their speech is virtually always intelligible and they can sequence well-formed sentences into narratives. They are able to use language to name, classify and reason. They can also use language in sophisticated ways: to establish dominance, to taunt, tease, soothe and to give or hide information. In school, they continue to learn about subtleties of meaning (you can write with a pen and a pig can live in one) and implied requests ('I think its time to clear up' really means 'Put those toys away now!'). Primary school children may be learning up to eight new words a day.

Language is both public and private. Vygotsky (1962) described how language is gradually used internally to think.

Language skills continue to increase into adolescence; complex vocabulary and sentence structures are acquired, and such language skills contribute to literacy. Reading provides opportunities to learn new words and grammar. In the teenage years, language is important for reflecting on the rules of interaction, expressing emotions and accepting ambiguity. There are marked sex differences in language skills at this stage, and, of course, teenagers communicate less with their family and more with their peers. Peer culture is created through shared language, and language skills are vital for establishing and maintaining relationships. Creativity and humour in language is most marked in adolescence, where new words and new uses of old words serve to identify social groups and exclude non-members. There is also an increase in understanding of idioms such as 'get a grip'. At the same time, most teenagers are adept at switching 'codes' so they can have conversations with their grandmother, teachers and friends in acceptable ways.

Language learning is a continuous, lifelong process; it is never finished.

How does language develop?

Language acquisition depends on children being exposed to language. Children who are deprived of language in their environment have serious communication difficulties (Kreppner *et al.* 2007). It is clear that children learn language in a social context, but the speed at which they do so has led some to suggest that a special capacity drives the process, sometimes known as the 'Language Acquisition Device'. However, computer modelling shows how grammar and vocabulary can be learned from the environment and how there tend to be rapid increases of learning (such as the vocabulary and grammatical explosions). Neuroscientific evidence shows that language processing can occur elsewhere in the brain if the usual processing areas are damaged in childhood, which makes it seem unlikely that certain parts of the brain are specialised for language development before it begins.

Babies and young children are very keen to communicate. As adults try to work out what children want to say, they provide a rich language environment.

Although exposure to language is important, language acquisition is not just about imitation. Children say things that they are unlikely to have heard, such as, 'I gived it'. Some would argue that such creativity is due to an innate understanding of how language works, or more likely, children look for patterns and find them in language.

The environment into which we are born shapes our genetic communication potential. It may also be that learning the form, content and use of language is influenced by the environment and genetic factors in different ways.

Language loss in dementia may give some clues to how components of communication are separate. Grammatical skills can remain long after the words that make up the sentences cease to be meaningful, so people can construct sentences but not remember or understand the words in them.

CHILD DIRECTED SPEECH

There is something special about the way people talk to babies and children. Language directed at children tends to consist of short, simple sentences presented at a slow pace. It includes lots of repetitions and is at a higher pitch than usual. These variations on adult speech change in response to the child's perceived developmental level, and in response to the child's reactions. This modified language has been described as 'child directed speech' or CDS (Snow 1972). There is also a type of CDS used in signing families, where the signs they use are more exaggerated for a baby.

Babies do seem to prefer to listen to CDS, especially when it expresses more positive emotion than other adult speech (Singh, Morgan and Best 2002). CDS seems to help children recognise that this speech is meant for them. It might also help them recognise when it's their turn to speak, as there is often a rising intonation at the end of an adult's turn. In addition, CDS can help them focus their attention on something else that the adult is talking about (Dominey and Dodane 2004). CDS is particularly important for language development because it seems to make it easier for children to hear the gaps between words (Thiessen, Hill and Saffran 2005), which otherwise come in a continuous stream that can be hard to interpret.

Adults respond to children's speech in various other ways which help them learn language. Children use an assortment of clues to work out what words mean; what they can see, hear and feel, the words others use, and the social situation, and of course adults provide many of these clues. Children with more gestures early on have parents who gesture more, and they grow up to have larger vocabularies (Meredith, Rowe and Goldin-Meadow 2009).

'Recasting' is where an adult repeats what a child has said, in a more adult form; for example, 'He comed' might be responded to with 'Oh, he *came*, did he?' Similarly, 'expanding' would be responding by saying, 'Did he come on Saturday?'(Saxton, Backley and Gallaway 2005). Parents do this when their children's language development is slower (Girolametto *et al.* 1999), but obviously less often as there is less to expand. Adults are also good at naming things that children are interested in, including their own and others' thoughts and feelings, thereby developing better social understanding. Most importantly, the amount of time an adult and child are focused on and talking about the same thing influences the child's later language development, in addition to the child's ability to share attention (Markus *et al.* 2001). Three-year-olds who have long conversations and reading sessions with adults have larger vocabularies and better understanding of language than those who do not (Beals, DeTemple and Dickinson *et al.* 1994). However, those with better vocabularies and understanding of language would be able to have longer conversations, so it is difficult to disentangle causal relationships. Nonetheless, adults help children learn language when they follow the child's lead and talk about what they are interested in.

'Teacherese' (Robb *et al.* 2003) is a style of adult interaction which seems to help children take part and learn more; it includes responsiveness, fun and turn-taking, similar to CDS.

RESPONSIVE INTERACTIONS

The way adults talk to children may not be as important as whether or not they are responsive to the child's attempts to communicate. The emotional availability of a significant other is a factor in a child's language development; it is responsive interactions which are important (Pressman *et al.* 1999).

Newborn babies are inclined to watch faces, and their eyes can just focus on a face when they are held in someone's arms. When infants hear a voice, they increase their scanning of a face, particularly the eyes. Even newborn babies are keen to communicate. They can imitate facial expressions and use these skills not just to respond to adults but also to start interactions (Nagy and Molnar 2004). In a responsive interaction, adults notice and respond to cues from a baby, often with delight. Those babies who get positive responses to their attempts to engage and vocalise do more of it. They realise they can have an effect on people. They want to share their thoughts and feelings and understand those of others; this is known as 'primary intersubjectivity' (Trevarthen 2001). From about two months of age, babies and responsive adults can engage in 'proto conversations' using facial expression and noises. Thus the babies learn the basics of turn-taking and understanding facial expression. More than this, such exchanges and being 'in tune' is pleasurable for both parties. The hormone oxytocin is released when we are with someone we care for, and higher levels of it help us understand others' thoughts and feelings better (Domes *et al.* 2007).

At first, babies like to be copied in interactions; after about three months of age, they enjoy slight changes in the response from another. After about six months of age, babies use a range of sounds to communicate and express emotions which can be recognised by caregivers and which are used in co-operative interactions (Papaeliou, Minadakis and Cavouras 2002). It is important to note that no interaction is perfectly responsive; the best only achieve it about 30 per cent of the time. But the babies and children keep trying until they achieve the response they were after (Tronick 2007). By a year old, children are not only responsive to people but they actively attempt to share their interest in something with others.

Peer interactions are important in language development, too, as a source of 'socio-cognitive conflict'. In other words, peers won't always agree, providing opportunities to learn the language of negotiation and problem-solving. In some cultures, children interact with just a few caregivers; in others, many. Some people value independence and others interdependence; all of these factors affect children's interactions and therefore their language development.

Children's temperament is also relevant here, as it will affect their attention skills, what they respond to and to what degree. Children have their own language-learning styles, and those whose early language is more socially oriented learn emotion words more readily than those whose early language is more object-related. Predictably, extraversion seems to be linked to the development of good language skills. Temperament also has an effect on how rewarding interactions are with the child, and therefore how much they occur.

Emotional development

To some extent, emotional development seems to be innate, but as with language development, environmental factors are also relevant. Emotional development is complex and rapid. Emotional skills emerge early and are largely developed before a child goes to school.

We all develop primary emotions: disgust, happiness, anger, sadness, surprise and fear, and this process starts very early. Babies less than a week old can distinguish happy, sad and surprised expressions, and they may try to imitate them. By 11 weeks old, babies are affected by their mother's facial expressions: they freeze in response to fear and show interest in response to a happy face. At three months of age, babies react positively to positive speech and negatively to negative talk, so even though they don't understand what we say, they understand the meaning of intonation. By the age of two, children can talk about emotion in themselves and others, and they can change how they feel through things like comforting themselves or teasing others. At this stage, toddlers begin to understand that behaviour relates to feelings: that crying might mean someone is sad and that hugs can make people feel better. By five, children can work out how external events have affected others' emotions, for example that someone might be sad if their hamster has died. Children at this age may still be confused when verbal and non-verbal cues are at odds with each other, however; for example, someone saying they feel fine when they look ill.

Through their school years children get better at managing their emotions, so they are not just immediately expressed. They become aware of the rules in their culture about which emotions can be expressed, in which contexts and how. They learn how to cope with difficult emotions by rationalising or minimising them. Between seven and ten years of age, children develop an understanding of mixed and ambivalent feelings. Displays of empathy increase, especially in children from families which discuss the complexity of feelings, are empathic and which have clear behaviour boundaries. At about age ten, children begin to take control of their feelings and take responsibility for their behaviour. Children who use more emotion words (Fabes *et al.* 2001) and who are better at managing their own emotions and understanding other people's feelings are more popular.

During adolescence, young people develop a sense of identity, and there is a 'psychosocial moratorium' (at least in Western societies) while they do this. In other words, there is a recognition that adolescence can be an emotionally difficult time. In early adolescence, massive changes occur in the organisation of the brain. This phase has been described as 'starting the engines without a skilled driver' (Dahl and Spear 2001, p.69), because emotions surge ahead before the thinking, organising and control parts of the brain are mature.

Teenagers become sophisticated at describing their emotions, interpreting social situations and regulating their emotions accordingly. They are also acutely aware of how the ability to control their feelings affects peer approval. There are gender and cultural differences regarding which emotions are expressed and how, which are refined in adolescence. During this time, young people develop an increased ability to mask emotions as well as an ability to use emotion to manage relationships. And, as if we didn't know, teenagers experience more negative moods and more mood swings.

Emotional literacy

Emotional literacy describes the skills which help us to understand and manage our own and others' emotions. Key skills are often described as:

- knowing how we feel
- knowing how others feel; empathy, sympathy
- labelling how we feel
- understanding that emotions aren't always expressed accurately
- coping appropriately with emotional situations, managing/ changing our feelings and those of others
- using emotions to assist thought, motivating oneself, delaying gratification.

It may also be important to include other skills such as attention to emotions, emotion repair and adaptive disclosure of emotion.

Our emotions affect everything we do and influence the way we think. Emotional literacy skills seem to be linked with success in a number of areas. In particular, an optimistic thinking style has positive effects on academic performance, productivity at work, satisfaction in interpersonal relationships, coping with stress, reducing vulnerability to depression and better physical health (Seligman 2006).

How do emotional skills develop?

ATTACHMENT

At birth human babies want to make strong emotional bonds with another person initially in order to stay safe. This drive to connect with a caregiver is probably what lies behind much language and emotional development. Newborn babies show signs of distress in response to an uncommunicative face (Nagy 2008).

Anxiety triggers the need for affection, comfort and safety, and a baby seeks close contact with a caregiver. The caregiver's response to this is crucial to the child's emotional development. A soothing response to distress will enable the baby or child to calm down. They can then spend time and energy on play, exploration and learning. Other, non-soothing responses can have long-term negative consequences for the child's development.

Ainsworth *et al.* (1978) describes a secure attachment as a relationship where caregivers respond to a child in ways which are predictable and comforting; they provide sensitive responses to their children's communications and emotions. Most importantly, this results in interactions which are pleasurable for caregiver and child; smiles and laughter maintain and develop the relationship, as with any relationship. It is also important for adults to recognise when a baby or child no longer wants to interact, or is tired and wants to stop.

If securely attached children are distressed, they know they will receive help and comfort. Negative emotions are also met with a sympathetic response, which then allows the child to begin to tolerate these feelings, and to make sense of them and the situation that caused them. Securely attached children learn that they can communicate their feelings and their thoughts and that this will lead to predictable and desired outcomes (Crittenden 1995), because they are listened to, understood and responded to. Being understood in this way strengthens the attachment further.

Attachment shapes one's expectations of people. A securely attached child will expect positive interactions with others. Factors within the child are relevant, as we all have different temperaments from birth. Unsurprisingly, children with difficult temperaments elicit more negative interactions, and those with easy temperaments receive more positive responses. Preschool children who are securely attached are more sociable and empathic towards others; they are also less hostile and anxious and have more social support and resilience than those who are not. They also have more complicated make-believe play. These children are more likely to be liked and to have successful relationships when they are older. Children who are securely attached understand emotions better than those who are not (De Rosnay and Harris 2002). Securely attached children also have better language skills; it seems that attuned or responsive interactions help babies learn about both language and emotions. Where there is a secure attachment and mothers stimulate and respond to their babies, language skills develop well (Murray and Yingling 2000).

The reverse is also true. Gesten *et al.* (1986) found that securely attached toddlers used more complex language than cognitively matched, maltreated children did. So a secure attachment can facilitate language development, and language is important in developing and strengthening attachments. Through language, carers can reinforce important messages such as 'I will come back'. Meins *et al.* (2001) found that the degree to which mothers talked about their child's thoughts and feelings at six months related to their security of attachment at a year old.

A secure attachment confers considerable resilience to adversity and enables children to grow up to be effective and positive parents themselves. Through attachment babies learn the skills to be co-operative, collaborative, communicating people (Fonagy 2003). However, only about 60 per cent of us are securely attached. An insecure attachment might make life more difficult, but it can often be overcome. Children who have initial insecure attachments can go on to form secure attachments later on.

Various adults can also become attachment figures as children get older, including, most importantly, teachers (for some children they might be the first secure attachment figure). This doesn't mean children stick to such adults as limpets, but that children can recognise them as reliable sources of information and support.

EMOTIONAL COACHES

It seems that adults want to teach, and children are inclined to learn from those they trust. How do adults help children understand the emotions they are experiencing? They often respond to the baby's or child's emotion by matching their facial expression, perhaps adding some exaggeration, to separate it from their own emotions; this is known as 'markedness'. Then they might suggest a verbal label, like 'That's sad', and perhaps offer ideas about emotion regulation ('Would a hug help?'). So adults are emotional coaches using language.

Adults also help children learn about what they and others think and feel by being 'mind-minded'. This means they talk to a baby assuming he or she has a mind, even before it is fully formed. This happens when they treat the child as intentional through meaningful interpretations of early vocalisations. In other words, the baby makes a gurgle and the caregiver responds with, 'Are you hungry?' Thus babies develop the ability to understand their own and others' thoughts and feelings because adults treat them as if they already have these skills. This helps children recognise their own feelings, learn what to do about them and understand them in others (Fonagy and Target 1997). Adults who talk to children about their own and others' thoughts and feelings have children who have a better understanding of what others might think or feel, or a better 'theory of mind' (Peterson and Slaughter 2003).

Children and young people talk to each other and learn from each other more and more as they grow up. Their conversations with each other are different from those with adults; they talk about thoughts and feelings more with other children than with their parents, and even more with friends (Brown and Donelan-McCall 1993). Kopp (1989) also observed that children talk about feelings in pretend play with others, and through this they begin to understand more about how to deal with feelings, especially difficult ones.

It is important to remember that it takes two to make an effective responsive interaction. A parent's ability to be mind-minded and provide emotional coaching is related to the quality of attachment and the child's ability to think about others' thoughts and feelings, as well as the development of their own language skills.

Babies clearly have feelings and take part in social interactions before they develop spoken language, and both interactions and emotions play a part in language development. However, it seems that an urge to communicate and link with others underlies much of child development. As children get older, what they want to communicate is less likely to be obvious from the context, so they need language to share their thoughts and feelings.

Language, thinking and emotional development intertwined

Children learn about communication, emotions and thinking at the same time. They rely on people they trust for information about the world, what things are called, how people are feeling and what might happen next. This relationship with others also helps them develop skills such as executive function, the ability to control and regulate other abilities and their behaviours (Carlson 2009). As others provide emotional and language coaching, children learn about people and how to interact with them. Language, thinking and emotional skills are necessary to engage with the coaching others want to provide children, and these skills continue to develop through such conversations.

Emotional, linguistic and cognitive growth influence each other, but it is difficult to tease out how this happens. For example, language development seems to be more advanced when a child has good attention control and more positive emotions (Dixon and Smith 2000). We also know that children with strong attachments develop better thinking, attention and language skills (Robinson and Acevedo 2001), and that there is also a correlation between emotional understanding and verbal ability (Bastian, Burns and Nettelbeck 2005). It is easier to play and chat with someone who is calm, talkative and attentive, so we can understand how such children get more learning opportunities. But were these children always easy to interact with, and is that why they developed well? Or did they gain these advantages because they were coached by responsive adults?

Bloom and Beckwith (1989) suggest that the rate of a child's language development is strongly influenced by his or her emotional state. The two-year-olds they studied could not communicate verbally when they were upset or excited. Therefore, Bloom and Beckwith argue that the rate of early language development is related to the amount of time a child spends in a calm state. So situations of great anxiety or excitement might impair language development, particularly if they are prolonged. Even as adults, language processing is affected by our emotional state: if your feelings match the language you hear, it is easier to understand (Glenberg *et al.* 2009).

Perhaps the most obvious link between emotion and language is that language is important for expressing and regulating thoughts and feelings. Although we can think non-verbally, we tend to think about how we feel and share our feelings in words. A child's ability to understand language predicts how well he or she understands emotions (Pons *et al.* 2003). Children who can understand and talk about emotions are better able to deal with them, because emotional regulation is, at least in part, dependent on the development of thinking and language skills (Thompson 1991). An example of how this works is that children's ability to distract themselves in a frustrating situation seems to relate to their language ability (Stansbury and Zimmermann 1999). These children may say things to themselves like, 'It doesn't matter, I can do something else'.

Language can provide a moment of contemplation between the experience of an emotion and its expression. Language plays an important role in self-regulation, and children who have some control over their emotions are more predictable, less intimidating and more popular. From around the age of six, thinking in words has become habitual, as has an increasing ability to reflect on and plan sequences of actions. Children of this age also begin to consider multiple consequences of actions, and part of any consequence is consideration of the emotions their actions provoke. In adolescence, multiple perspectives can be considered simultaneously, which requires complex language, emotional and thinking skills. Language development is therefore crucial for reflection and a key part of developing sophisticated emotional and thinking skills. The increasing need for sophisticated language development has far-reaching consequences, because children who can control their attention and behaviour are likely to be more popular and do better academically (Eisenberg *et al.* 2004).

Children also learn about themselves in conversation, especially when they have conversations about past experiences and, with help, develop 'personal narratives'.

Brain development

Language and emotional development, and indeed the development of thinking, depend on the growth of the brain, which quadruples in size during childhood.

Babies use their brains differently to adults. They seem to use what will become their language-processing areas to help them understand faces (Tzourio-Mazoyer *et al.* 2002). This might explain why focusing on faces is important for social interaction and learning language. Also, areas of the brain important for joint attention seem to be working when children are processing words (Mills, Coffey-Corina and Neville 1994). Imaging studies of the brain give us insights into how parts of the brain work together; in early development, parts of the brain involved in understanding people and social interaction are closely linked to those involving emotion (Grady and Keightley 2002); self-awareness and awareness of others are also closely linked in terms of the brain areas involved, particularly the right medial prefrontal cortex.

The social brain – essentially the frontal lobe – is underdeveloped at birth, but it develops as children learn the language and culture of the people around them. External influences can affect the way the brain develops. Connections in the developing brain are pruned or strengthened depending on how much they are used, so the environment, particularly early interactions, can affect brain structure and function (Gerhardt 2004).

This rapid growth in the brain, combined with observations about the rate of language learning in childhood, has led to ideas about critical periods in development. Before computer modelling of language learning it seemed that there was a critical period for learning language before adolescence. In other words, if language has not developed in childhood then it is unlikely to; however, the situation is not as straightforward as this. It is certainly true that young children learn new languages (including sign languages) faster than older children or adults. Also, evidence from studies of brain damage affecting language show that before ten years of age children are likely to recover their language but after 12 only 60 per cent recovered language. However, language learning does continue into adolescence and beyond, into adulthood (Nippold 1998). Recent computational models (Seidenberg and Zevin 2006) also suggest that there isn't necessarily a biological or chronological limitation on language learning, but that language stops when it is finished. The more we learn about the brain, the more it seems that the brain's potential to develop is unlimited. So although early brain growth is important for language and emotional development, such development can occur in later years.

Cognitive skills

Cognitive or thinking skills can also influence the development of communication and emotional skills. For example, much early interaction is dependent on the development of the infant's ability to share attention. That is the ability to focus on what someone else is looking at, so that the infant and caregiver both give attention to the same thing. A baby's early abilities to detect eye direction, emotion and intentions allow the child to develop shared attention, which then helps the development of theory of mind (Baron-Cohen and Belmonte 2005). Shared attention is a deceptively simple skill, but if it is not in place, interactions will be impaired. Toddlers with autism have difficulty with joint attention, making it hard for them to develop language and social understanding (Mundy and Neal 2001). Babies who are better at following their parents' eye gaze at six months of age have better vocabularies at two; visually impaired children have fewer words for specific objects. It is important for a child to realise that when they point at something, the adult will look and think about the same thing as they are, which is often a very positive experience. By 12 months, babies point to things to share information with others. It's not just shared attention that is key, but also that both individuals know they are sharing something. This is known as 'secondary intersubjectivity'

(Trevarthen 2001). Shared understanding is the basis of all interactions and communication.

Other cognitive skills such as memory and attention are necessary for language development, particularly those which affect the ability to process speech. In order to learn language, it is essential to be able to listen, remember, process and gain meaning from what others say. Babies who have difficulty processing rapidly presented sounds are at great risk for later communication problems (Benasich *et al.* 2006).

The vocabulary spurt coincides with a development in the child's ability to categorise objects: recognising, for example, that cows, sheep and pigs somehow go together. Another example of language and thinking developing in concert is when a child realises that something still exists although it can no longer be seen; this is called 'object permanence'. At the same time as babies understand this, they use the word 'gone' a great deal.

Theory of mind

A theory of mind helps us understand what other people might be thinking and feeling, as well as reasons for their behaviour, both of which influence how we interact with them. We recognise when someone is not listening to us, or when they are excited, pretending or being silly, and we react accordingly. While we assume that others think and feel, we have no direct evidence of that, which is why it is called theory of mind. Theory of mind is necessary for us to interact well with others and seems to be heavily influenced by language development.

The presence of a theory of mind can be shown in the 'false belief task'. In the false belief task, a child sees another person witness a toy being hidden. Once this person has left the room, someone else moves the toy. The child's task is to say where the original witness *thinks* the toy is, not where it is now. The child is only able to do this if he or she appreciates that the person who left the room did not see the toy being moved. The child has to realise that another person's experiences are different from his or her own. Children before the age of about five and those with autism will assume that the person who left the room knows that the toy was moved, even though they can't have seen it happening, because that is what the child knows. Autistic children have difficulty developing a theory of mind and therefore assume that others' experience is the same as their own.

Recently it has become more obvious that even young babies have some ideas about others' intentions and therefore the beginnings of a theory of mind. For example, one-year-olds got angry when adults *refused* to give them a toy but did not get annoyed when they *couldn't* do so (Behne *et al.* 2005). Interestingly, theory of mind and empathy may well use overlapping parts of the brain; clearly, it is difficult to develop empathy if you have no notion that others also think and feel.

Fonagy *et al.* (2004) see theory of mind as something which develops out of attachment and which helps us to understand ourselves as well as others, and therefore strengthens and maintains attachments. We know that adults being mind-minded helps develop theory of mind (Meins *et al.* 2002), but specifically how often parents ask children to reflect on the other person's feelings after a conflict also seems to be important.

The development of theory of mind is closely linked with verbal ability (Hughes *et al.* 2005; Pyers and Senghas 2009). As children acquire a theory of mind, their understanding of mental-state words develops, and they are more likely to refer to the thoughts and feelings of their friends and siblings (Patnaik and Babu 2001). Emotional vocabulary is necessary to understand others' feelings, as is the ability to understand sentences such as 'If you do Z, they feel Y'. Also, language skills are needed to have conversations with others about feelings, and to consider what other people might be thinking and feeling. Through the development of a theory of mind, children can also learn more language because they infer from others' behaviours what they are referring to and what they might mean by an unfamiliar word.

Older siblings and friends can help in the development of theory of mind through fantasy and pretend play. However, children need to be able to use and understand complex language to set up and join in such pretend play.

Play and interaction

Play and interaction are important in the development of emotional, thinking and communication skills. There are opportunities to rehearse scripts relating to real life and be creative to make up their own. Play is a way of finding means to express emotions, letting off steam, and learning adult roles and is important for language development, especially narrative skills. Through play, children learn about the use of symbols; toys represent real things. Language develops hand in hand with symbolic play, so children who link words also link sequences of pretend play. Pretend play, with accompanying talk, may help discussions of emotions such as fear and anger, which could be difficult in other contexts (Haight and Sachs

1995). (Truly 'free play' may be less available to some children in Western culture because adults feel they need to teach and provide educational toys (Hirsh-Pasek and Michnick Golinkoff 2003).)

Interaction with peers is crucial for emotional and language development and vice versa. Peers often provide both models for language and 'problems' to solve where language skills come in useful and can be refined. Collaborative learning (Rogoff *et al.* 2003) is where children do meaningful things in collaboration with more skilled 'teachers'; this is effective because children are doing things which are useful and interesting to them.

Social interaction is therefore important for the development of many skills relevant to language and emotional development, such as turn-taking and considering others' points of view, but it also requires skills in these areas.

Conclusion

Language and emotional development occur together and affect each other powerfully. Both language and emotional development can be influenced by the environment and, in particular, the relationships between carers and the developing child. Individual differences within children also affect the way their language and emotional skills develop. Complex skills such as co-operation, self-control and language are learned through interactions with a caregiver, usually before the age of five (Kaiser *et al.* 2000). If these are not in place, much subsequent development is jeopardised.

Chapter 2

The Links Between Emotional and Behavioural Difficulties and Communication Problems

Are there links between communication problems and SEBD?

The development of communication, emotional and thinking skills is a complicated, intertwining process, so it isn't surprising that problems can occur and difficulties in any area can influence the development of the others. What has become more and more apparent is that communication and social, emotional and behavioural difficulties often occur together. This means that anyone working with children with SEBD should consider the possibility of their also having communication problems. When working with children with communication problems, one should be alert to the possibility of SEBD or mental health issues. Before considering the reasons for this co-occurrence, it is important to clarify what is meant by communication problems and social, emotional and behavioural difficulties.

Defining social, emotional and behavioural difficulties

The term 'social, emotional and behavioural difficulties' encompasses many different kinds of problems. There are various definitions and classifications used by different disciplines; those who work in health and education may use different terms to describe similar problems faced by young people. The major issue with defining and diagnosing social, emotional and behavioural problems and mental health issues is that the process is largely subjective. 'Deviance, like beauty, is in the eye of the beholder' (Bennett 2005, p.11).

THE MENTAL HEALTH PERSPECTIVE

One definition of mental health problems is:

> Mental health problems may be reflected in difficulties and/or disabilities in the realms of personal relationships, psychological development, the capacity for play and learning, and in distress and maladaptive behaviour. They are relatively common, and may or may not be persistent. When these problems are persistent, severe and affect functioning on a day-to-day basis they are defined as mental health disorders. (DH 2004)

The International Classification of Diseases (World Health Organization 1996) has the following diagnostic categories for child mental health disorders in children and young people:

- hyperkinetic disorders, including ADHD

- conduct disorders. These are the most common: 'Typical behaviour includes unusually frequent and severe temper tantrums beyond the age that this is normally seen, severe and persistent disobedience, defiant provocative behaviour, excessive levels of fighting and bullying, cruelty to others or animals, running away from home and some criminal behaviour.' (BMA Board of Science 2006, p.5)

- mixed disorders of conduct and emotions, e.g. conduct disorder and depression

- emotional disorders with onset in childhood, e.g. anxiety phobias and depression

- disorders of social functioning, e.g. selective mutism, attachment disorders

- tic disorders, e.g. Tourette's syndrome

- others, including stuttering (although other communication difficulties are considered to be disorders of psychological development).

In America, the Diagnostic and Statistical Manual of Mental Disorders, 4th edition, or DSM-IV (American Psychiatric Association 1994), provides similar categories.

Other relevant aspects of the child's life, such as medical conditions, environmental stresses and specific delays in development can be included in the DSM-IV or ICD classification, in what is known as a 'multi-axial scheme'. There are six axes in ICD-10:

- Axis One: Clinical psychiatric syndromes, e.g. conduct disorders
- Axis Two: Specific disorders of psychological development, e.g. disorders of speech and language
- Axis Three: Intellectual level
- Axis Four: Medical conditions, often associated with mental and behavioural disorders
- Axis Five: Associated abnormal psychosocial situations, e.g. significant stress in the family
- Axis Six: Global assessment of psychosocial disability, e.g. How well are they able to function at school/home?

(World Health Organization 2007)

To capture a holistic view of a child or young person, the World Health Organization also has the International Classification of Functioning, Disability and Health, which aims to provide a view of difficulties from a biological, individual and social perspective. It doesn't just consider the medical diagnosis but also the effect the diagnosis has on what the person can do and the degree to which this affects their participation in society. This view also takes personal and environmental factors into account. So two children with the same diagnosis can be affected in different ways, and their progress will be affected by their personality and the environment in which they live. We need this level of detail to understand and support young people with complex issues surrounding communication and behaviour.

Nearly ten per cent of children aged 5–16 have a mental health disorder. Mental health issues are more likely in boys than girls, and boys are more likely to have conduct disorders and ADHD, whereas girls have more emotional disorders, such as depression or anxiety (Office for National Statistics 2005).

In the UK, children and young people who have social, emotional and behavioural difficulties are not always referred for a psychiatric assessment, nor are they necessarily given clear diagnoses like those in DSM-IV or ICD-10. This may mean that some children and young people don't get the help they need. However, it is not clear the extent to which the 'medicalisation' of something like conduct disorder is useful. The ICD-10 and DSM-IV categories are descriptive and therefore subjective; they are not based on theories of why these things occur, so even if young people have the same symptoms of conduct disorder, these may have occurred for widely differing reasons, and this wider context should not be overlooked. The multi-axial classifications are supposedly useful for guiding treatment, gathering information and for research. However, some suggest they hamper research because they categorise those with similar symptoms together rather than considering causes. Another issue with these classifications is that they don't differentiate those who perhaps experience the world differently because their brains are 'wired' differently; for example, in autism spectrum disorders (ASD; also known as autism spectrum condition) and in those who suffer because of external events such as post-traumatic stress disorder (PTSD), both are considered to have mental health disorders.

THE EDUCATIONAL PERSPECTIVE

The Department for Education and Skills (2001) *Special Educational Needs Code of Practice* describes behavioural, emotional and social difficulties (BESD) as:

> a learning difficulty where children and young people demonstrate features of emotional and behavioural difficulties such as: being withdrawn or isolated, disruptive and disturbing; being hyperactive and lacking concentration; having immature social skills; or presenting challenging behaviours arising from other complex special needs. Learning difficulties can arise for children and young people with BESD because their difficulties can affect their ability to cope with school routines and relationships.

A more recent definition is:

> The term 'behavioural, emotional and social difficulties' covers a wide range of special educational needs (SEN). It can include children and young people with conduct disorders, hyperkinetic disorders and less obvious disorders such as anxiety, school phobia or depression. There need not be a medical diagnosis for a child or young person to be identified as having BESD, though a diagnosis may provide pointers for the appropriate strategies to manage and minimize the impact of the condition. (Department for Children, Schools and Families 2008a).

According to the Office for National Statistics (2005), children with an emotional disorder were twice as likely to have special educational needs (SEN) as those with no emotional disorder, and half of those with conduct disorder had SEN. Children with social, emotional or behavioural difficulties in school are seen as having SEN if additional or different educational arrangements are needed to support them.

In effect, the term 'social, emotional and behavioural difficulties' encompasses children and young people who may not have very much in common: those whose behaviour is unacceptable, those who are under stress, those whose brains are different as well as those who are mentally ill. There are low levels of agreement on who has SEBD; because adults expect different standards of behaviour and have varying degrees of tolerance and skill in dealing with behavioural issues, different contexts place different demands on children and young people, and the quality of relationships vary. There are also cultural differences and variation in what parents and teachers see as problem behaviours.

Children and young people who have externalising difficulties (including disobedience, aggression, delinquency, temper tantrums and overactivity) (mostly boys) are more likely to be referred for extra help, while those with primarily emotional or internalising difficulties (mostly girls) may not be identified as having problems. However, the 'emotional' part of the definition is very important: to consider the behaviour alone ignores the reasons why it may occur. Unacceptable behaviour leads to negative responses from others, which can further lower self-esteem and add to emotional difficulties. Basically, these are children who are both troubled and troubling, and they often don't receive the services they need to address their social, emotional and behavioural difficulties.

Defining communication problems

There are various ways of defining and categorising communication problems. Although there are broad categories of communication problems included in the ICD and DSM categorisations, such as expressive language disorder (problems expressing yourself), receptive language disorder (difficulty understanding language) and stuttering, these definitions fail to capture the complex nature of communication difficulties. The use of such broad categories may have made it more difficult to find links between communication difficulties and social, emotional and behavioural problems.

There are many types of communication problems. There may be problems with the larynx, leading to harsh voice quality. Sometimes there are difficulties with the muscles necessary to produce speech, which can lead to slurred speech. Alternatively, children may have difficulty using the sound system of a language, so many two-year-olds may call the sun a 'dun', but if this pattern persists, the child may need help. There is also verbal or articulatory dyspraxia, a disorder of planning, where the messages from the brain are 'scrambled', leading to difficulty co-ordinating the muscles for speech.

Sometimes a communication problem is described as a language 'delay' because the course of typical development is followed but at a later age than is usually the case. A language disorder occurs where the course of typical development is not followed, though in practice, language delay and disorder often occur together. Some children have what is termed a 'specific language impairment' (SLI), where language difficulties seem to be the primary issue, and development in other areas may be relatively unaffected. Some children and young people are described as having pragmatic language impairment because they have difficulty using language appropriately to interact. This can be a difficulty in its own right, or it can arise because of difficulties with form and content which disrupt interactions.

It is more likely that a young person with communication problems will be male, although that could be because communication problems in girls are under-detected (Tomblin *et al.* 1997). Communication problems are not only many and varied but they can change in nature over time. Some children have transient language delay, and some have communication problems which persist throughout their lives.

It is possible to have difficulty with the form, content or use of language or, indeed, all three. Most young people with communication problems have patterns of difficulty that are quite individual. Some examples of communication problems are listed below. The more areas involved, the less likely is a good outcome; this is particularly the case if the child or young person has difficulty understanding language.

Difficulties with form:

- speech that is difficult to understand
- problems discriminating speech sounds, so 'catch' and 'cat' might sound the same
- using sentence structures more appropriate for someone younger, e.g. 'me got them', at four years
- problems linking sentences with words such as 'and', 'but', 'so', 'then', etc.
- difficulty sequencing sentences to make a meaningful narrative.

Difficulties with content:

- problems learning new words
- difficulty retrieving known words at the right time, also known as 'word finding' difficulties
- limited vocabulary for emotion words.

Difficulties with use:

- limited eye contact and problems with other aspects of non-verbal communication
- poor turn-taking and difficulties with starting and ending conversations
- problems 'repairing' when two people talk at once or misunderstand each other
- unable to understand or respond to feedback from the listener
- unable to stay on topic in conversation
- problems with verbal negotiation or conflict resolution.

Difficulties with understanding language

- difficulty understanding complex sentences such as passives, e.g., 'The boy was kicked by the girl'. Since the first person mentioned in a sentence is usually the one who is active, someone with communication difficulties might think the boy did the kicking
- difficulty understanding idioms such as 'get a grip'
- being unable to identify the key theme or topic.

See Appendix 1 for a more detailed list of behaviours which could indicate that a child or young person has communication problems.

Communication problems and social, emotional and behavioural difficulties often occur together

Research over many years has found that children who have communication problems are likely to go on to develop social, emotional and behavioural difficulties, and sometimes mental health disorders (Lindsay, Dockrell and Strand 2007). Over 50 per cent of children who have communication difficulties develop SEBD and mental health difficulties of all kinds. This means they are three to four times more likely to develop such difficulties as other children.

It is also the case that between 60 and 95 per cent of children and young people with recognised SEBD or mental health issues also have communication problems which may go unrecognised (see Chapter 3).

Not only do social, emotional, behavioural and communication difficulties often occur together, but the association seems to start early. Cohen and Mendez (2009) studied preschoolers who had behavioural issues and found that they were also likely to have difficulties understanding language and regulating their emotions. These children were from low socio-economic groups, and their ability to interact with others remained poor or declined over the year they were studied.

Are there links between particular SEBDs and specific communication problems?

The short answer to this is probably not, or at least they haven't yet been identified. One reason why finding such links is difficult is the way in which SEBDs are identified and measured, and who identifies them; for example, parents and teachers often have different perspectives on a child's behaviour. Communication problems are difficult to assess, and the choice of assessments in research obviously influences what is found. There are some reports that communication problems seem to link to delinquency in boys but not in girls, but this conclusion depends on who you ask to rate behaviour (Brownlie *et al.* 2004).

Botting and Conti-Ramsden (2000) assessed over two hundred children with communication problems and found that those with complex language problems (i.e. difficulty understanding language and expressing themselves) were most likely to have a clinical level of behavioural difficulty. It may also be the case that those who do not understand language are more likely to withdraw (van Daal, Verhoeven and van Balkom 2007). There seems to be an association between difficulty understanding language and aggression. Young people who do not understand what others say to them feel frustrated and inept, and they might respond aggressively (Sigafoos 2000).

It seems that the strongest link between behaviour problems and communication difficulties is where the child or young person has pragmatic difficulties or problems with the use of language. The risk of these children having behavioural issues, such as hyperactivity and a lack of skills to join in with others, may be four times as high as for those with other communication difficulties (Ketelaars *et al.* 2010).

The types of behavioural issues may change over time: in young children with communication problems, the most likely behavioural difficulties seem to be related to hyperactivity and attention (Lundervold, Heimann and Manger 2008.) Groups of children initially identified as having communication problems first showed behaviours indicative of frustration but later experienced more anxiety, lower self-esteem and tended to withdraw (Haynes and Naidoo 1991; Rutter and Mawhood 1991).

There are many potentially confounding factors, one of which is gender. De Bellis (2003) suggests that maleness is a risk factor for stress-related vulnerability. As we have seen, boys are probably more likely to have communication difficulties and SEBD.

So, as Lindsay *et al.* (2007) point out, there are no straightforward links between communication difficulties and behaviour problems, but rather a complex interaction between factors within the child and environmental factors.

Why do communication, emotional and behavioural problems occur together?

There are many potential answers to this. There may be different links for different groups of children: perhaps something different is happening for those who start out with communication problems and then develop SEBD, compared with those who have behavioural and perhaps undetected communication problems. There may also be different links at different stages of a child's development.

The next sections will consider the possibilities. Do communication problems cause SEBD? Could social, emotional and behavioural difficulties cause communication problems? Perhaps some children and young people are unlucky enough to experience both, and these two problems are not linked. There are also of course factors which could cause both SEBD and communication difficulties.

It is also important to remember that not all children with SEBD have communication problems, and vice versa.

Do communication problems cause social, emotional and behaviour difficulties?

There is certainly evidence that children with communication problems often go on to have behavioural or mental health difficulties, but it is not clear that there is a causal link.

Longitudinal studies show that those who have communication problems, especially problems understanding language, often go on to develop mental health difficulties (Lindsay *et al.* 2007; Snowling *et al.* 2006).

At least one study has found a modest correlation between vocabulary and violence in 19-month-old children (Dionne *et al.* 2003); and children with hearing loss have behaviour problems which vary in severity in relation to their language skills rather than their hearing loss (Stevenson *et al.* 2010).

It is possible to identify at-risk children early on. Children who have problems developing language at ten months old are more likely to have mental health difficulties at one and a half (Skovgaard *et al.* 2008), and children with communication problems at age five are at much greater risk of social phobia in adolescence (Voci *et al.* 2006). The risk of developing SEBD or mental health difficulties increases when children also have general learning difficulties and severe language problems.

Some would argue that the behaviours of children with communication difficulties are adaptations to their language limitations rather than behaviour problems per se (Redmond and Rice 1998). In other words, children with communication problems are likely to be less responsive to language and initiate less than their peers, as well as less likely to rely on adults to help out where they are unable to negotiate verbally. These behaviours can be interpreted as immaturity or anxiety, misinterpretations which are discussed further in the next chapter. It is undoubtedly the case that children with communication problems are often misunderstood and seen as solely immature or as behaving inappropriately.

HOW COULD COMMUNICATION PROBLEMS LEAD ON TO SOCIAL, EMOTIONAL AND BEHAVIOURAL DIFFICULTIES?

We have all experienced frustration over not being able to get our message across, so it is possible to understand how this frustration might lead to behavioural outbursts. Caulfield (1989) tested this 'frustration' hypothesis by giving children who had communication problems a task that was particularly taxing for them, a naming task. Predictably they were more likely to misbehave when faced with such a task. Similar situations frequently occur in classrooms where children with communication problems are unable to meet the language demands of the lesson. As the difficulty of the curriculum increases, so does the stress on those who don't have the communication skills to access it; this often leads to 'off-task' behaviour which gets children and young people into trouble.

Children with communication problems, especially those which have not been recognised, are often misunderstood. The difficulties they have with understanding what people say and expressing themselves can be misinterpreted as non-compliance. If the child were trying their best but still got told off, behaviour problems could result. Also, children who don't understand what others say can misinterpret intentions and get confused and angry.

LANGUAGE IS IMPORTANT FOR REFLECTION AND SELF-CONTROL.

As language is a set of symbols for reality, it gives some distance and the possibility of reflection. Language enables us to reflect on feelings and events, and this helps us understand ourselves and other people. This reflection happens though self-talk (where we describe what we're doing and think out loud) and then internal speech (where we talk to ourselves, in our heads).

Words provide a moment of thought and delay in which unpleasant feelings can be handled in ways other than denial or immediate action, so they also help us gain some control. We use words to distract ourselves, to think about causes of unpleasant feelings and to calm ourselves. Words are also the way we can share and learn coping strategies, such as, 'I go for a walk if I'm upset'. When strong emotions are given verbal labels, the emotions become more manageable, and this can be seen through neuro-imaging (Lieberman *et al.* 2007).

Self-reflection and self-control are key components in successful social problem-solving, which is being able to think of solutions to issues such as such as 'someone has the toy I want'. The development of emotional regulation in early childhood is interrelated with emotional understanding and language skills (Eisenberg *et al.* 2004), and limited language is linked to poor self-control (Beaver *et al.* 2008). Children with SLI have been shown to have a delay in development of emotional knowledge (Brinton *et al.* 2007). Having the language skills to think about experiences helps us to develop the self-control and self-organisation which is known as executive function (Winsler, Fernyhough and Montero 2009). Communication problems are associated with boys' difficulty with emotion regulation, even for boys with age-appropriate abilities in other areas (Fujiki, Brinton and Clarke 2002).

Another reason children with communication problems might develop social, emotional and behavioural difficulties is that they miss out on, or are even excluded from, opportunities to interact with other children. Children learn to interact well through interacting with others, but communication problems can impact on the ability to interact successfully. Children with communication problems are less likely to try to join in with play or start a conversation; they are also less able to respond when other children ask them to join in (Irwin, Carter and Briggs-Gowan 2002). Failure in social interactions can lead to a loss of confidence, self-esteem and willingness to try again. Children with communication problems are often rejected by others and even bullied or scape-goated (Conti-Ramsden and Botting 2004). This can initiate a negative spiral of interactions where the child with communication problems finds it increasingly difficult to interact in a positive way (Rice 1993). Interaction skills and acceptance by peers seem to relate to a child's success in school overall.

There is therefore some evidence for ways in which communication difficulties could lead on to social, emotional and behavioural difficulties, even mental health problems, given the social problem-solving difficulties and isolation they can lead to (Zadeh, Im-Bolter and Cohen 2007). However, there are always children and young people with communication problems who do not develop SEBD, so there is no straightforward link. Some children may benefit from protective factors in their environment, fewer learning difficulties and less severe communication problems.

One major implication is that in many children with 'behavioural' problems, communication difficulties are primary and their remediation could ameliorate the behavioural difficulties. Identifying and understanding communication difficulties is a first step (see Chapter 4). Simple measures can make a great deal of difference. Reducing the linguistic complexity of speech when speaking to children with communication problems can also result in positive behavioural changes (Prizant et al. 1990).

It is important to add that bilingualism per se is not a risk factor for communication or behavioural problems. In typically developing children, bilingualism confers considerable advantages, not least in terms of an awareness of language as an abstract entity. However, learning an additional language is most successful when the child can engage in frequent conversations with native speakers, so any child who has difficulty engaging with others will be at a disadvantage. Therefore children who are having problems developing communication skills or who have developmental delays or neurological difficulty may experience problems when learning additional languages, which could result in emotional and behavioural difficulties.

Do social, emotional and behaviour difficulties cause communication problems?

Social, emotional and behavioural difficulties might result in withdrawal, which could in turn lead to reduced opportunities for participation and fewer opportunities to learn how to interact. Thus problems with emotional development could limit language development. However, there is little evidence for primary mental health difficulties leading on to problems with communication. Not all children with SEBD go on to develop communication problems, and some would argue (Stringer and Clegg 2006) that, apparently, secondary communication difficulties in SEBD exist because of late identification of pre-existing difficulties.

Early communication difficulties are often the first indication of other developmental difficulties such as problems with learning or mental health.

Many social, emotional and behavioural problems co-occur with communication problems

Many childhood mental health conditions have communication problems as part of the diagnosis or as a commonly occurring feature.

ATTENTION DEFICIT HYPERACTIVITY DISORDER

Attention deficit hyperactivity disorder (ADHD) is the most common mental health difficulty (MHD) in childhood. ADHD occurs when a child has poorer attention than you would expect for his or her age, and is also impulsive and hyperactive. This poor attention, impulsiveness and hyperactivity is so severe that ADHD causes significant problems with interactions and learning. ADHD is easy to confuse with other difficulties: inattention can also be characteristic of PTSD, attachment disorder, oppositional defiant disorder, conduct disorder, learning difficulties and neurological dysfunction.

ADHD is also the MHD most commonly associated with communication problems. Love and Thompson (1988) found that about 75 per cent of children with language delay also had attention deficits. Forty-five per cent of children with ADHD have also been found to have communication difficulties (Tirosh and Cohen 1998). Children who have ADHD have often had delayed language development, and they may have residual expressive language difficulties and problems understanding language. At least some children with ADHD have processing difficulties similar to children with SLI (Cardy *et al.* 2010) and those who have SLI and speech sound difficulties seem to be at greater risk of ADHD (McGrath *et al.* 2008). Children and young people who have ADHD often find it difficult to organise their ideas into a coherent narrative. Many of them also have difficulty with the use of language (Bruce, Thernlund and Nettelbladt 2006). For example, these children do not always respond to questions or requests and are likely to interrupt others. They also give less feedback in conversation and have difficulty monitoring the listener's understanding of what they have said. They also seem to find it difficult to alter their communication style in response to the speaker or the situation.

Many of the difficulties that children with ADHD have are associated with executive function: the way the brain organises itself, plans what to do and what not to do and where to focus attention. Being able to use inner speech is important for this and many children with ADHD do not have inner speech (Reck, Landau and Hund 2010). This means that they cannot use language effectively to plan a course of action, but also that all their thinking will be verbal, which can be very annoying for people around them. Other difficulties associated with executive function deficits are: not being able to stay on topic, interrupting, and saying too much. Also the impulsivity that these children experience means that they often have to rephrase because they haven't thought through what they are going to say.

A child's ability to concentrate is, of course, vital for other learning: good attention at four and half relates to all sorts of later positive academic outcomes including language development (NICHD 2003).

Therefore, it is possible that for some children, social, emotional and behavioural problems and communication difficulties stem from the same cognitive deficit, in the case of ADHD, executive function problems

CONDUCT DISORDER

Children and young people with conduct disorder (Gilmour *et al.* 2004) and oppositional defiant disorder often have difficulties with the social use of language, for example with staying on topic, negotiation and understanding other people's non-verbal cues (Audit and Ripich 1994). Those with conduct disorder may also have difficulties with theory of mind, or at least identifying facial expressions (Sharp, Fonagy and Goodyer 2008).

AUTISM SPECTRUM DISORDERS

Those with ASD experience difficulties in communication, mainly in terms of its use rather than its form, social interaction and stereotypical behaviour. Some of the differences associated with ASD can be described in terms of problems with empathising, but also include the potential strengths of a greater tendency towards systematising, shown sometimes in repetitive or narrow interests (Baron-Cohen 2009). The communication problems children and young people with ASD experience vary widely. All children with ASD have problems with the use of language, but some have problems with the form and content of language like those in SLI (Lindgren *et al.* 2009). Indeed, the links between autism and communication problems imply that there is perhaps a shared genetic basis for them. For example, young people who have a history of SLI are at a much greater risk of ASD than other children (Conti-Ramsden, Simkin and Botting 2006). There is also evidence that relatives of children with autism are at an increased risk of communication problems (Tomblin, Hafeman and O'Brien 2003).

SELECTIVE MUTISM

Selective mutism may seem to be an example of a mental health difficulty leading to communication difficulties, though causation is often more complex than this. It occurs where a child finds verbal communication difficult in one or more situations while being able to communicate well in other environments. Often, selective mutism begins when a child starts school and the child does not talk in school, or in the presence of unfamiliar people, although they have no difficulty talking at home amongst their family. Children who develop selective mutism often have a history of anxiety in social situations. Once a child has been unable to speak at school for a while, the pattern is often difficult to break.

Children who are selectively mute often have language delays, too (Cohan *et al.* 2008), so it is not clear whether the emotional difficulty is primary. It seems that these are children who are prone to anxiety, and their communication difficulties make them more sensitive to verbal interactions, which can lead to mutism in some settings. In addition, there is often some kind of emotional risk factor in children who are selectively mute (Champagne and Cronk 1998), such as attachment difficulties or emotional or physical immaturity, which might also lead to communication problems.

POST-TRAUMATIC STRESS DISORDER

PTSD can disrupt communication and attention. Reminders of the traumatic event can trigger a limitation of the capacity to use words, as well as impair attention and memory. Children can show symptoms such as sleep problems, hypervigilance (being 'on guard') and aggression. They may find it difficult if their routines are disrupted and they may play repetitively, acting out what they have experienced. Children who are traumatised find it difficult to put their thoughts into words or organise coherent narratives. Overall, children who have more PTSD symptoms tend to have a lower verbal IQ; it is not clear if this is because having better verbal skills is protective, or if PTSD reduces verbal capacity (Saltzman, Weems and Carrion 2006).

More significantly, there may be a permanent change in brain chemistry, or even brain structure, in children due to ongoing trauma such as abuse or neglect (De Bellis *et al.* 2002b; Perry *et al.* 1995). If trauma is persistent, then the fear state it produces also becomes persistent, resulting in a child who is hypervigilant, focused on threat-related cues (which are mainly non-verbal), anxious and impulsive. These behaviours may be useful in a threatening situation, but not once it has passed. Hypervigilant children find it difficult to learn and interact, and it seems likely that this will have significant negative effects on their development in all areas. Therefore, PTSD is a psychiatric problem which could potentially impair both communication and emotional development. A healthy attachment can protect a child from the worst effects of trauma because the child has a basic sense of trust, has learnt some self-soothing and can look to caregivers for comfort. Conversely, children with poor attachment may be affected more severely.

TOURETTE'S SYNDROME

Tourette's syndrome is characterised by tics, which are involuntary, rapid, repetitive movements. Tourette's is diagnosed when such tics persist for more than a year, before adulthood. Initially they are non-verbal, but later verbal tics appear as well. Verbal tics include: explosive repetitive verbalisations, throat clearing and grunting, and they may be obscene in nature. Verbal tics can certainly impair interaction, although children with this syndrome often have relatively intact communication skills. Some children with Tourette's syndrome have communication problems such as trouble formulating sentences and using abstract language, which could be caused by the same executive function difficulties which leads to this disorder (Legg *et al.* 2005).

SCHIZOPHRENIA

Schizophrenia is rare and those who experience it have two or more of the following features: disorganised thinking, delusions, hallucinations, very disorganised behaviour and low mood. Onset is usually in adolescence or early adulthood. Individuals who go on to develop schizophrenia often have delayed language development (Mouridsen and Hauschild 2008).

In schizophrenia, thought is affected; but thought processes are expressed through language. Scans suggest that differences in language processing areas underlie thought disorder (Sabb *et al.* 2010). So is it possible to tell the difference between disordered language and disordered thought? When a child's sentences are not clearly organised or linked together, this can be seen as a symptom of thought disorder, but this is also seen in children with communication problems where it is viewed as a linguistic/structural deficit. This underlines the importance of a good differential diagnosis, not only for potentially schizophrenic children but for all children with social, emotional and behavioural problems in addition to communication difficulties.

DEPRESSION AND ANXIETY

Children who have anxiety and depression are also likely to have communication difficulties. The communication problems are often with the social use of language: sometimes children who are seen as 'shy' are actually lacking in communication skills.

So communication and mental health difficulties often co-occur, and in many mental health conditions the first sign of difficulty is that language is slow to develop (Hagberg, Miniscalco and Gillberg 2010). Difficulties with the use of language are common in mental health conditions.

Common causes of social, emotional, behavioural and communication problems

As has been shown, there is limited evidence for simple, direct links between social, emotional and behavioural difficulties and communication problems. There are, however, various factors which could be responsible for both kinds of impairment, including, as we have seen, executive function limitations. Genetic predisposition, adverse environmental factors, interaction and attachment problems, child abuse and learning difficulties are all potential causes of both emotional/behavioural and communication difficulties which will be considered in the next section.

GENETIC PREDISPOSITION

There is little evidence for single genes having a significant effect on language or behaviour; it seems more likely that many genes have small effects in combination with environmental influences. It is rare for specific genes to be solely responsible for particular conditions; for example, the same genes may influence the language difficulties in SLI and ASD.

Studies of identical twins seek to disentangle the effects of genes and the environment, although the assumption that twins experience exactly the same environment and upbringing can be challenged. The twins early-development study (Oliver and Plomin 2007) has followed the development of 1300 pairs of twins. The results suggest that the same genes are responsible for learning ability and disability, but that their effects are small. It seems that genes can have some general effects and that the environment has more specific effects on children's development. The same study found that associations between verbal and non-verbal ability and behaviour were modest, although the link may be stronger in those who have difficulties.

As regards communication skills and difficulties, the main influence on language (vocabulary and grammar) seems to be the environment, but genes are more influential as regards speech (Hayiou-Thomas 2008).

The genetic influence on behaviour problems seems to be similarly balanced by environmental factors, and it is likely that the genetic contribution is from many genes. There may be more of a genetic influence for severe behaviour problems, but this is controversial. Genetic factors can lead to a susceptibility to developing a mental health disorder, but only in the presence of other environmental factors; this could be the case in depression, schizophrenia and ADHD.

What this means is that some children have a genetic predisposition that, in a challenging environment, could lead to a variety of difficulties likely to include social, emotional and behavioural difficulties and communication problems.

DISRUPTION OF EARLY INTERACTIONS

It takes two to interact, and sometimes early interactions are not successful because the parent or child (or both) are unable to be communicative or responsive. Some parents find it easier to interact with their babies and children and to interpret and respond to what they are trying to say than others. Even newborn babies notice when interaction is not going well (Nagy 2008), and this will affect their interest and confidence in subsequent interactions. Most babies and children are keen to interact from birth and have the skills to do so, but this is not always the case, and then adults may have to work extra hard to have a responsive interaction. Stresses on either the parent or the baby or child can also make it difficult to have a relaxed conversation.

The stress of parenting should never be underestimated; babies need intensive and relentless amounts of care, which can put a strain on anyone. As they grow older, children may need less intensive attention, but their needs are always changing and throw up new challenges. The quality of the interactions a child experiences affects their language development, especially the degree to which adults are able to be sensitive to the child and the quality of the reciprocity. Positive interactions also help children develop positive behaviours (Denham, Renwick and Holt 2008).

Depressed mothers (or fathers) are unable to be sensitive to their child's needs, or to respond positively to them. They are also less able to do so as their children get older and more demanding, as they have fewer resources to draw on. Consequently, language delay in children is associated with maternal depression. This lack of stimulation also affects other areas of development, so children whose mothers were depressed when they were less than a year old are more likely to have learning difficulties. Babies of depressed mothers may learn to tune out female speech but will listen to male speech (Kaplan, Dungan and Zinser 2004).

Another factor which can affect interactions is the temperament of those taking part. Babies and children who are inattentive, impulsive and distractible may be more difficult to interact with, so from very early on they may experience fewer positive interactions.

Children who have communication problems will similarly be less responsive and may eventually have fewer opportunities to learn how to interact because of this. These children may find social interaction stressful and unrewarding, which can lead to depression and withdrawal, and in some cases they become less playful and compliant. The adults in these unrewarding exchanges also suffer frustration and can become discouraged; mothers of such late talkers reported more parenting stress (Irwin *et al.* 2002). Other children can be reluctant to interact with those with communication problems because their attempts to have conversations or play are unsuccessful.

Similarly, children with SEBD tend not to elicit as many positive interactions from their caregivers as other children, which can also lead on to language delays and compound their behavioural issues. Children with behavioural difficulties tend to elicit directive, less-responsive interactions from adults. Unrewarding interactions can influence our feelings about a person, and so a negative spiral can begin. Negative perceptions of each other influence negative behaviour between mothers and sons (MacKinnon-Lewis *et al.* 1992), and where mothers had negative attitudes towards their six-month-olds, the children were more likely to have behaviour problems at four years of age (Bor *et al.* 2003). The relationship between parenting styles and children's behaviour may be bi-directional, so that a child's behaviour can lead to a deterioration in the supportiveness offered by parents (Huh 2006), undermining the idea that poor parenting 'causes' poor behaviour. It may be that the 'connectedness' between carer and child is an important factor in the links between language and behaviour. Where it occurs, the child is not only learning useful skills but also 'being kept out of trouble' (Brophy and Dunn 2002).

So anything which reduces the quality of interactions between a child and their carer can have an impact on further interaction, communication and the development of positive behaviour.

ATTACHMENT DIFFICULTIES

Ainsworth *et al.* (1978) proposed three types of mother–child attachment, (though these can be applied to whoever is the principle caregiver). There are caregivers who respond to children in ways that are predictable and comforting, leading to secure attachments. To achieve this, parents have to be aware of their child's emotions, be able to tolerate them and able to help the child feel calmer, or cheer the child up as necessary. In other words, they are emotional coaches. Children who have secure attachments learn that they can get help and support if they need it. However, if parents have not had an emotional coach themselves, it is very difficult for them to take this role for their children.

Insecure attachments also occur. There are caregivers whose responses are predictable and distressing, and there are those whose responses are unpredictable and inconsistent. These respectively lead to anxious-avoidant and anxious-ambivalent types of attachment in children. There are also children who have disorganised attachments, often in abusive or neglectful situations, where the children are torn between needing affection from their caregivers and being frightened by them. These children may seem depressed, irrational and disorganised and are very likely to have social, emotional and behavioural difficulties. They are likely to be hostile, violent and controlling when they reach school age. Such children are also liable to have experienced deprivation.

Anxious-avoidant children learn that expressing their feelings leads to uncomfortable outcomes, for example parental anger, rejection or unavailability. Therefore, such children will try not to express their feelings; to them, only thinking is meaningful. These children may be hostile and socially isolated. They may seem calm but their heart rate, when measured, shows their high level of stress. Anxious-ambivalent children learn that expressing their feelings has no predictable outcome, so for them neither emotions nor thinking is particularly meaningful. Attachment difficulties and the great stress they cause children can affect their ability to think and learn. These children may be over-dependent and lack confidence and therefore be less likely to engage in the play and exploration which is important for their development. They may also be very focused on behaviour rather than language, because what they have been told has been unreliable. In an insecure attachment, stress and fear can inhibit the parts of the brain that are important for understanding other people. This is how insecure attachments do damage. In the NICHD study (2003) 90 per cent of those whose mothers rated them as having behaviour problems had attachment difficulties.

As children grow older they don't necessarily have to be near a parent to feel safe, but they remember how this relationship has made them feel, so they are gradually able to become more independent and self-confident. Regrettably, the same is true of an insecure attachment: it is remembered and affects future interactions. Thus early attachment difficulties can affect children's abilities to form attachments as they grow older and reach adulthood. Insecure attachments have negative effects on children's social, emotional and communication development as well as their ability to learn. However, having an early attachment difficulty does not mean that a child can't form secure attachments in later life.

The child's role in forming an attachment should not be underestimated. Some children, for example those with ASD, find it harder to interact regardless of how sensitive and responsive their parents' interactions are.

Attachment difficulties often impact on communication skills; for example, insecurely attached children learn fewer words for thoughts and feelings (Lemche et al. 2004). Parents of insecurely attached children may not help their child develop clear narratives about their lives, experiences and feelings, and the inconsistency they experience can result in illogical thinking and confused narratives. Differences in the language abilities of violent and nonviolent individuals reflects the importance of attachment for brain development (Fonagy 2003).

ENVIRONMENTAL FACTORS

Unfortunately many children have to deal with adversity of various kinds, sometimes from before birth. The following are all possible risk factors for developing language and social, emotional and behavioural difficulties: learning difficulties, sensory impairment, central nervous system dysfunction (such as cerebral palsy), adverse family conditions, low socio-economic status (SES), psychosocial stress, parental (particularly maternal) mental illness, perinatal complications, brain injury and premature birth. The more of these factors that are present, the higher the likelihood of impaired language, emotional and behavioural development.

Some of these factors, such as prenatal exposure to drugs and alcohol can directly affect a child. Foetal alcohol syndrome seems to increase both the likelihood of communication problems (Thorne and Coggins 2008) and mental health difficulties such as ADHD (Elgen, Bruaroy and Laegreid 2006). Prenatal cocaine use also seems to have a negative effect on language development (Bandstra et al. 2002). Other factors are likely to stress the family and reduce the likelihood of the positive interactions necessary for development. For example, parents may be less responsive to their infants in overcrowded environments (Evans, Maxwell and Hart 1999).

CHILD ABUSE AND NEGLECT

When parent–child interaction breaks down to the extent that child abuse or neglect occurs, there are obviously negative effects on many areas of a child's development. Abuse and neglect have a harmful effect on a child's general development, health and growth, including their emotional, cognitive and linguistic progress. Language development may be more affected than some other areas of development because it is more environmentally sensitive. The emotional effects include the development of a negative self-image, difficulty managing emotions and behaviour problems.

Abusive and neglectful mothers interact with their children less; they are unlikely to play with or talk to them and more likely to ignore what they say. The language they do use tends to be more controlling. Similarly children in such situations are less likely to interact with their carers.

For a baby or child, not having their basic needs met, which is what happens in neglect, is intensely stressful. In addition to nutrition and other physical care, a baby needs help to be calm in a world that makes little sense to them and can therefore be terrifying.

The prefrontal lobe, or social brain, develops largely after birth; this is an advantage in that we can learn the language and culture we are born into and, indeed, the sort of attachment formed prepares us for the environment we grow up in. The disadvantage is that neglect can severely impair the development of the social brain, in particular the capacity for empathy, as well as the total size of the brain (De Bellis *et al.* 2002a). Children who were neglected in orphanages in Eastern Europe had very limited language and social skills (Rutter *et al.* 2007). Where there are pleasurable interactions between carer and baby the frontal lobe develops; the reverse is also true (Gerhardt 2004). Perry *et al.* (1995) suggests that children who are chronically abused are in a hypervigilant fear state where they are so focused on non-verbal cues that they are unable to pick out verbal information which will enable them to learn language.

Abused children are not good at recognising emotions in others and they are unlikely to express their own emotions verbally. They find it difficult to consider contextual cues when interpreting emotions, and they have particular problems interpreting complex and conflicting emotions, so they may think that others are being aggressive towards them even when they are not (Pollak *et al.* 2000). They are also at a disadvantage in learning how to manage their own behaviour because they do not have the appropriate emotional vocabulary. Such children have difficulty making and maintaining relationships and learning. There could also be long-term effects, considering a history of abuse and neglect is common in adults who have psychiatric difficulties.

Neglect has the most significant effect on language development because of the lack of positive responsive interactions. Children who have been abused and neglected have mostly been found to have difficulties with expressive language when they are younger. During middle childhood, they seem to have difficulty with the abstract and pragmatic aspects of language as well as expressive and receptive delays (Rogers-Adkinson and Stuart 2007). Their communication problems also seem to increase over time (Hooper *et al.* 2003).

However, it is not always clear which is cause and effect when it comes to abuse and neglect and developmental difficulties. A complex pattern of factors seem to contribute to the language delay commonly seen in neglected children. The child's ability to learn, the mother's experience of abuse and neglect and her lack of acceptance of her child are all relevant (Sylvestrea and Mérettec 2010). Children who already have neurological or developmental difficulties, such as communication problems and who are also subject to social stressors, are more likely to suffer child abuse. As well as this, child abuse and neglect can be seen as the result of many factors, one of which is the child's tendency to health and developmental problems, including communication problems, and the stress this creates. It may also be that the same factors which lead to child abuse contribute to the development of disabling conditions such as conduct disorder and learning difficulties (Spencer *et al.* 2005).

Disability makes abuse easier, especially in children who are communicatively impaired. Their communication problems also make it harder to identify that abuse has taken place, and such children may not be seen as competent witnesses.

COGNITIVE LIMITATIONS, LEARNING DIFFICULTIES AND PROBLEMS WITH EXECUTIVE FUNCTION

Learning difficulties, general neuro-developmental delay or difficulties in specific areas such as executive function or information processing may be common causes of behavioural and language problems.

Children with learning difficulties are more likely to develop mental health problems than other children (Emerson and Hatton 2007). A third of children with learning difficulties will also have a mental health disorder, especially ASD (Emerson and Hatton 2007). The likelihood of learning difficulties is greater when children have more than one 'disorder' (known as 'co-morbidity'), and a third of children using mental health services have multiple disorders (Office for National Statistics 2005).

Specific deficits in cognitive processing could underlie some behavioural and language difficulties and explain why these are often closely associated. Cognitive processing is defined as the skills required for problem-solving and abstract reasoning. These skills include processing speed, memory and attention, and deficits in these areas could impair both behavioural and language functioning, as it includes the speed at which children process emotion cues (Rock, Fessler and Church 1997).

Executive function is the organisation of other functions such as attention and memory and includes the use of inner speech to self-regulate. Executive dysfunction has been linked to learning disabilities, antisocial behaviour and communication problems. As we have seen, executive dysfunction is also implicated in ADHD, Tourette's and autism.

Children with SLI have been shown to have difficulties with auditory processing (Archibald and Gathercole 2006) and executive functioning (Hughes, Turkstra and Wulfeck 2009), particularly attention. Hughes *et al.*

(2000) found associations between poor verbal skills, antisocial behaviour, violent pretend play and poor executive function: a combination that's difficult to unpick.

Neuro-developmental delay is implicated in some language delays (Buschman *et al.* 2008) and behavioural problems. However, it can only provide a partial explanation for the co-occurrence of communication and behaviour problems, as not all of these children also have learning difficulties.

DEVELOPMENTAL EFFECTS

To add to the complexity, the links between social, emotional and behavioural difficulties and communication problems change over time. The foundations of emotion, language, thinking and behaviour skills are laid down in a child's early years. As each of these develop, or fail to, they can affect the development of other areas. Preschool children with communication problems are likely to have immature and overactive behaviour. After starting school, they may go on to develop internalising disorders, particularly anxiety. Later on, into adolescence, externalising behaviour problems may occur, particularly if there have been literacy difficulties.

Children and young people also respond to their difficulties in different ways. They may make accommodations to problems and later on may attempt to overcome or mask them.

Conclusion

There are likely to be various links between communication problems and SEBD (see Figure 2.1). No one link is relevant to all children with SEBCD. Some children are resilient. There are children with communication problems and no behaviour difficulties, and vice versa. Similarly, there are children who live in adversity and who do not develop emotional or communication problems. However, for some children, multiple factors seem to conspire against typical development and their impact is strongest where positive interactions are rare.

Although attachment disruption may be a significant factor, it is important not to ignore the wider context, particularly where that includes psychosocial disadvantage. The mediating factor in the development of some communication, emotional and behavioural problems seems to be differences in thinking, either in executive function or theory of mind, which have direct effects on interactions, thereby influencing further learning and social adjustment.

More subtle measures of communication skills and behaviour will be necessary to identify any relationships between the two more clearly. There is also a great need for more research in this area. It is therefore important for practitioners to consider *both* the communication skills and the emotional and behavioural difficulties a child may experience.

As there is lots of co-morbidity between developmental disorders (Dyck and Piek 2010), it is probably better to identify each child's strengths and needs than to try to identify a specific problem. It is also useful to gather information about other significant risk factors impinging on a child, as well as to note their strengths using a classification such as the ICF (see Chapter 5 for more details); this may help us understand more about how some children and young people experience social, emotional, behavioural and communication difficulties.

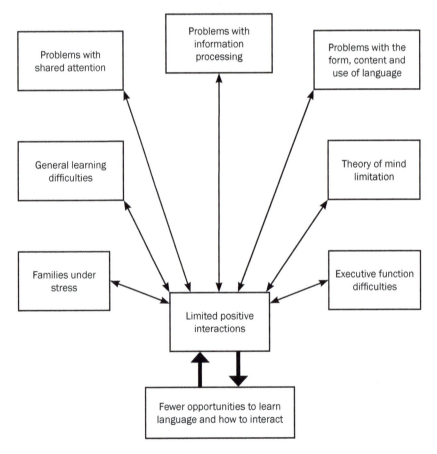

Figure 2.1 Possible links between SEBD and communication problems

Chapter 3
Undetected Communication Problems and Their Impact

In the last two chapters, I have argued that communication and emotional development are interlinked, so it is unsurprising that many children and young people have SEBCD. However, these links have not always been recognised and are still not obvious to everyone working with children who have SEBCD.

More seriously, there is a growing body of evidence showing that many children with social, emotional and behavioural difficulties have communication problems which have not been detected. The consequences of this are serious for the young people involved. They seem to be at greater risk of communication difficulties than other young people, and communication difficulties are often associated with serious negative effects on behaviour and emotional development, social interaction and learning. Young people with undetected communication problems are at risk of potential misdiagnosis and inappropriate interventions.

How many children have communication problems?
In order to appreciate the scale of communication problems amongst children with SEBD, it is important to appreciate how often communication problems occur in general. However, this is not straightforward. It is difficult to determine how many children in the general population have communication problems because various different definitions are used in research and practice by different professionals. This is illustrated by the many different terms used to describe sometimes-overlapping communication problems:

- specific language impairment
- speech and language delay
- delayed language development
- speech, language and communication impairment

- speech, language and communication needs
- speech, language and communication difficulties
- communication support needs
- developmental language disorder
- specific speech and language difficulties
- speech and language difficulties
- language disorder!

So clearly there is a problem with identifying how many children and young people have communication difficulties because there is no consensus on how to define them, and this is then compounded because the nature of communication problems seems to change over time. It is relatively easy to identify preschool children who are not talking as much as their peers, but as children mature, their language problems may appear primarily as difficulties with literacy, social relationships or learning. Also, young people may be reluctant to talk or interact, so any communication problems may not be apparent without specific investigations. Communication problems also become more or less obvious depending on the academic and social demands of the environment. A young person may cope well at home where the language is often predictable, and they may be perfectly able to have a conversation with their peers, but they may struggle in school where a different vocabulary is required, and the language is abstract and often refers to things beyond their experience. There may also be an unfamiliar style of conversation required in school.

Nonetheless, various studies have found similar incidences of communication problems in preschool children. Tomblin *et al.* (1997) sampled over seven thousand children in the United States and found a prevalence of SLI of 7.4 per cent. Law *et al.* (2000) found a figure of 5.95 per cent for speech and language delay in their review of the literature.

It has always been accepted that boys are more likely to have communication problems (and other developmental difficulties), but it may be that we have different expectations of boys and girls, so girls have to be more impaired before they are seen as having communication difficulties – or do they perhaps compensate more easily (Bleses, Vach and Lum 2010)?

There are also children and young people who have communication problems as part of another condition such as autism, hearing impairment, ADHD, dyspraxia or general learning difficulties. Furthermore, an estimated 1 per cent of children have the most severe and complex communication problems. These children and young people may have very little spoken language, serious difficulties understanding language, or be completely unintelligible and unable to indicate their basic needs, wants and desires when they begin school (Lindsay *et al.* 2008). So, overall it is estimated that about ten per cent of all children have some sort of communication problem. This is about the same as the number of children with dyslexia, and ten times the number who have autism (Bishop 2010).

Although there is little evidence about the prevalence of communication problems in school-aged children, there is evidence that language impairments can persist into adolescence and beyond (Clegg *et al.* 2005; Conti-Ramsden 2008; Whitehouse *et al.* 2009b) and difficulties with understanding language are most likely to persist (Clark *et al.* 2007).

In some parts of the UK, particularly in areas of social disadvantage, more than 50 per cent of children start school with communication problems (Locke, Ginsbourg and Peers 2002), and this research is beginning to be replicated elsewhere. Some of these children may 'catch up' with their peers; however, there is also evidence that these difficulties can persist and get worse (Locke and Ginsbourg 2003).

Perhaps all types of communication problems in children are on the increase. This is true in at least one Finnish town (Hannus, Kauppila and Launonen 2009). Many professionals who work with young children think there has been an increase in communication problems.

However, the number of children with SEBD and communication problems seems to be markedly higher: ten times higher than in the general population (Law 2005). Benner, Nelson and Epstein (2002) reviewed the literature on communication problems in children with SEBD and concluded that approximately three-quarters of children with SEBD also had language deficits and 'the rate of co-morbidity between language deficits and EBD tends to be stable or to increase over time' (p.7). More recent research confirms this (Benner *et al.* 2009). Also, as we have seen, children with communication problems seem to be at increased risk of social, emotional and behavioural difficulties (Durkin and Conti-Ramsden 2010; Lindsay *et al.* 2007).

Undetected communication problems in children with SEBD

There is some variability in the estimated level of communication problems in children with SEBD because of the different assessments used and different definitions of communication problems. Nevertheless, it is clear that children and young people with SEBD are at much greater risk of communication problems than the general population. There is also evidence that these communication problems are often undetected and unaddressed. Although many of the studies on undetected communication difficulties are small in scale, together they paint a worrying picture.

Undetected communication problems in children and young people with mental health difficulties

Over a long period of time, research has shown that a third or more of children referred for mental health issues have unsuspected communication difficulties (Cohen *et al.* 1998; Cohen *et al.* 1993; Cohen and Lipsett 1991; Giddan, Milling and Campbell 1996; Jones and Chesson 2000; Kotsopoulos and Boodoosingh 1987).

More recently there has been a focus on the nature of these communication problems. Earlier studies tended to focus on the form and content of language, but more recently there have been investigations into the role of the 'use' of language. Many children and young people with SEBD have difficulties with the use of language: the ability to use language appropriately to the person and the setting, understanding non-verbal communication and understanding implied meanings. Gilmour *et al.* (2004) found that two-thirds of children with conduct disorder had an unexpected social communication difficulty.

Undetected communication problems in early years settings

This is also the case in preschoolers. Schultheis (2001) analysed the language and behaviour of 129 preschoolers and found that children with behaviour problems were likely to have communication problems which were undetected.

Undetected communication problems in primary schools

A study of primary school children who were disruptive were found to be likely to have undetected communication problems, poorer social use of language skills and limited abilities to see others' points of view (Donno *et al.* 2010). It is also important to note that children who have reading difficulties are also at risk of having undetected communication problems (Nation *et al.* 2004).

Undetected communication problems in children in foster care

In a small study (Cross 2001), and in the intervening years, a large number of children and young people in foster care with the Integrated Services Programme have been found to have undetected communication problems.

Undetected communication problems in schools in areas of social disadvantage

A high proportion of children attending a mainstream inner-city secondary school were found to have difficulty understanding what they read. These pupils also had more limited communication skills (Myers and Botting 2008). Spencer, Clegg and Stackhouse (2010) reported on adolescents with undetected communication problems who attended a secondary school in an area of social disadvantage.

Undetected communication problems in those at risk of exclusion from school or excluded

Law and Sivyer (2003) found undetected communication problems in children with SEBD who had been excluded from school. This was also the case in Ripley and Yuill's (2005) study. Clegg et al. (2009) identified 10 of 15 boys at risk of exclusion from school as having previously undetected communication problems; however, they stress that the remaining five had good to above average communication skills.

Undetected communication problems in schools for children with SEBD

Studies have found that children with SEBD in special education have undetected communication problems (Burgess and Bransby 1990; Heneker 2005). One study showed that in a special school for children and young people with SEBD, less than half of the 74 per cent with language impairments had been detected (Stringer and Lozano 2007).

Children in residential care are also at risk. Hagaman et al. (2010) showed that 54 per cent of pupils had undetected communication problems, and that these students were not achieving as well as their peers academically.

Undetected communication problems in young offenders

More than 60 per cent of young offenders in one study (Bryan, Freer and Furlong 2007) had undetected communication problems likely to interfere with their rehabilitation. Further research across the world reports similar results (Snow and Powell 2008). Young people found to be responsible for a criminal act were no less intelligent than those not seen as responsible, but they had poorer vocabularies (Blanton and Dagenais 2007). Are those with undetected communication difficulties more likely to be criminally responsible, or just more likely to be judged so?

Studies of children and young people with SEBD of various ages, in differing contexts and using different assessments, have all found evidence of undetected communication problems. Current systems are clearly not effective at identifying communication problems in children with SEBD.

Why are communication problems often undetected?

Perhaps the main reason why communication problems are undetected is because they are not necessarily expected or sought out, but there are other reasons.

Lack of awareness and training

Although there has been progress in this area, professionals working with children and young people with SEBD or mental health difficulties are rarely trained in how to identify communication problems or indeed know how likely it is that communication problems will occur. Toppelberg and Shapiro (2000) suggest that child and adolescent psychiatrists need an understanding of language development and disorder in order to make the appropriate referrals. This is also true of any professional working with children with SEBD.

However, identifying communication difficulties is not straightforward. If you only talk to children and young people in informal situations, or briefly, it may seem appropriate or typical if they use few words or give less complex answers, or that you don't always understand each other. Some teachers, especially in secondary schools, have very few opportunities to have conversations with their students, so it's very difficult for them to judge how well they can communicate. Many children and young people have adequate communication skills in informal settings, but when more complex explanations or descriptions are required their communication skills fail them. In addition, there is some evidence that parents and medical professionals tend to overestimate the ability of children to understand language (Sattler, Feldman and Bonahan 1985), and these are the kinds of problems which often go undetected. All of this is complicated by some children's and young people's reluctance to communicate with adults. It is important to know what to listen for when considering a young child or young person's communication strengths or needs, and it is not a simple business; hence Chapter 5 on assessment.

Another relevant issue is that of co-morbidity, or how children with developmental difficulties often have more than one. For example, children who have communication problems are more likely to have developmental co-ordination disorder (DCD), also known as dyspraxia. There are overlaps between dyslexia and SLI, as well as speech sound disorders in children. SLI and ADHD also often occur together. In addition to this, it seems that children with SLI are at much greater risk of ASD. Sometimes systems do not reflect this co-morbidity, and professionals have to decide which is the primary or main difficulty. This may mean that the true complexity of a child's difficulties may be underestimated or unaddressed. It is often a mistake to think that the right label or diagnosis has been found for a child's difficulties and that other possibilities can therefore be excluded. As we have seen, it is often the case that a young person had communication difficulties *and* SEBD.

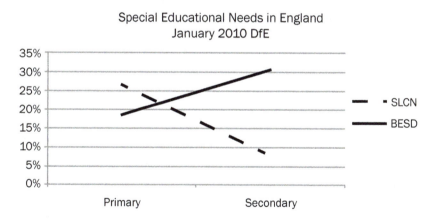

Figure 3.1 'Primary' special educational needs?

Co-morbidity is not always considered when trying to identify young people's needs. Figure 3.1 shows the number of children with communication problems (SLCN) and BESD in primary schools (5–11 years) and secondary schools (11–18 years) in England in January 2010. These figures are collected by the special educational needs co-ordinators in schools; they have to identify which is a child's primary need. The number of children with communication problems appears to plummet in secondary schools, while BESD rises sharply. Is this really the case, or are communication difficulties less recognised and supported in secondary schools? The linguistic and organisational demands certainly increase as children move into larger secondary schools and the curriculum becomes subject based; does this cause extra stress for those with communication problems, who then show behavioural difficulties? Is this an issue of co-morbidity where different aspects come to the fore at different times? Or is this all about becoming a teenager? What may be happening here is that communication problems that had been recognised are either resolved, which seems unlikely, or they are seen as less significant and perhaps are then less likely to be addressed. Or is this about children and young people who have communication problems being misunderstood or not getting access to the services they need?

Some say that there are no resources to meet these young people's needs, so there seems little point in identification. It is possible, though obviously regrettable, that the current situation of under-identification reflects resources rather than needs. Speech and language therapy services are rare in secondary schools and even rarer for children with SEBD or mental health difficulties. However, all professionals can use simple strategies to help to develop the communication skills of these children and young people (see Chapter 6).

Communication difficulties may be subtle

It is easy to recognise a child with unintelligible speech. However, children with SEBD are less likely to have these kinds of obvious communication problems. They are more likely to have difficulty understanding language, using it to express themselves and the social use of language. However, these sorts of communication difficulties can be difficult to spot. In particular it is difficult to identify when someone doesn't understand language; a child may not respond appropriately because they do not understand, but such a response might also be due to a lack of interest or co-operation. Young people, who do not always understand spoken language, may be unaware of this problem or unable to indicate when they don't understand. They may also have developed strategies to hide these difficulties, but as we shall see, this sort of difficulty with understanding language has many negative effects for a young person if it is not recognised and addressed. Again the answer to this problem is an increase in awareness of the possibility of communication difficulties and how they may show themselves.

Communication problems may be seen as behaviour problems

If a child or young person has communication problems, it will be difficult for them to understand what is expected of them, justify their actions, respond appropriately and interact with others without discord. If one is not aware that a child or young person has communication difficulties, such behaviours can seem like oppositional or at least unco-operative behaviour.

These are some examples of how communication problems are often seen as behavioural issues:

- children who don't listen or pay attention (because the language used is too complex for them to understand)
- children who don't do as they are told (because they don't understand what they have been asked to do)
- children who don't ask when they don't understand (because they don't realise they haven't understood or because they can't ask clarification questions)
- children who don't explain why they did something (because they can't easily construct sentences or narratives)
- children who interrupt or speak in an inappropriate way (because they are not good at 'reading' social situations or using the appropriate social communication skills).

Children and young people may be considered to have mental health difficulties because they have difficulty interacting with others or have difficulties expressing their ideas coherently; these could also be indicative of difficulties with communication skills.

Behaviour difficulties may be more obvious than communication problems

Communication difficulties may be overlooked if a child also has more obvious disruptive behaviour, especially if their communication problems are subtle. Although there does seem to be a link between communication problems and aggressive behaviour, it is obviously the aggressive behaviour which gets the urgent attention. Interventions to address behaviour may seem to be a priority, but these are unlikely to succeed if communication difficulties are not considered, particularly if these interventions are language based.

Psychosocial disadvantage

Cohen *et al.* (1998) found that children with undetected communication problems had mothers with less education than those children with typically developing language. One factor associated with good communication skills is supportive parents and, more importantly, a good school environment (Parsons *et al.* 2009). If these are not present, children's communication difficulties are unlikely to be identified and addressed. In the context of poverty and limited education, it is unsurprising that subtle difficulties such as communication problems are not detected or that help is not sought for them. Another issue relevant here is that communication problems may be detected but perhaps referrals are not made or appointments are not kept (Parow 2009). This implies that current services may not be flexible enough to support all children.

Chapter 4 will explore the links between language and social disadvantage further, but since we know the two are linked and that intervention can improve children's communication skills, services should be in place to identify and address children's communication problems in areas of social disadvantage.

Communication problems change in nature

Longitudinal studies, where children with communication problems are studied as they grow up, give us some insight into what might happen to others like them. However, the main finding of such studies is that outcomes are very variable – some do well and some less so – and we're not entirely sure why this is. Nevertheless, we do know that children and young people who have communication problems as they start school are at greater risk of literacy difficulties and limited social participation (Tomblin 2008). So if you met a young person later in their school career, it may not be obvious that communication difficulties underlie these problems. Their spoken language difficulties may seem to have resolved (although there may still be an impact on literacy) but often difficulties with understanding language and the social use of language remain.

Furthermore, as children reach adolescence the links between language and thinking become more apparent. As a child grows older communication problems impact on reasoning, organisation of knowledge and conceptualisation (Wiig 1995), so in adolescents communication problems can seem very similar to general learning difficulties.

The significance of communication problems

What might be persuasive in increasing the identification of communication problems is attention to the wide-ranging and significant implications they have. Communication problems have a negative impact on the ability to socialise and learn, and undetected communication problems can expose children and young people to misdiagnosis and inappropriate interventions as well as potentially exacerbating their social, emotional and behavioural difficulties. It is also important to note that outcomes for children with communication difficulties are very variable: some do well, some much less so.

Educational consequences

Children and young people who have communication problems are at much higher risk of difficulties with literacy than their peers (Tomblin 2008). Many of the skills necessary for literacy are based on spoken-language skills; so if a child has difficulty understanding what they hear, they will have difficulty understanding what they read. Also, children who find it hard to construct sentences or narratives when they speak are likely to have similar problems when they try to write. They might also have difficulty relating letters to sounds (Snowling and Hulme 2006). Even young people who have intelligible speech may have difficulty hearing the difference between speech sounds, segmenting words into sounds and blending speech sounds, which are all important skills for literacy. Good vocabulary skills are also crucial for reading, and children with communication problems are often at a disadvantage because even if they can 'decode' the letters into sounds, they may not recognise the resulting word. As most children mature, they learn more words and ways of expressing ideas and feelings through reading (Nippold 2007), so those who have literacy difficulties are excluded from further developing their communication skills.

Literacy problems can persist and even at the end of formal schooling, those with communication problems are likely to still need support for literacy (Snowling *et al.* 2006). Most seriously, a substantial minority of children with a history of communication problems are likely to be functionally illiterate (Tomblin 2008).

The frustration of falling behind one's peers with literacy and not being able to access learning in this way may be a link between communication problems and SEBD in some children (Tomblin *et al.* 2000). Most pupils in schools for children with SEBD have difficulty with literacy, and it is also worth noting that there is evidence of greater psychiatric difficulties in poor readers (Arnold *et al.* 2005). Literacy difficulties also seem to be a risk factor for social difficulties, unemployment and criminality. Female young offenders have vividly described the difficulties they have with listening, thinking, speaking and reading, and the problems it has caused them (Sanger *et al.* 2003).

However, literacy is not the only barrier to learning for children with communication difficulties. Most learning takes place through the medium of language. There have been recent attempts to increase the amount of dialogue in classrooms based on the premise that through discussion pupils can really understand concepts and develop their knowledge (Sheehy *et al.* 2009). Despite this, children and young people are still expected to listen for long periods of time in many classrooms. This could be an issue for many pupils (not least those with attention difficulties); however, if a young person has particular difficulty with auditory processing, learning in a mostly auditory environment is very difficult and stressful and many give up. Unfortunately, the social interaction and discussion that helps most children learn is in itself problematic for many children with communication problems. Communication problems can affect children's learning in other ways. Many words have two meanings; for example, we use 'mouth' for part of a person's face and the entrance to a river. We also use many terms for the same thing; for example, 'take away', 'minus' and 'subtract'. In addition to this, we may use the same phrase for something completely different, because a chicken curry can also be a 'take away'. So children with communication problems can be at a serious disadvantage in education.

The good news is that there has been some improvement in the literacy and educational attainment in more recent groups of children with communication problems (Conti-Ramsden et al. 2009). But still, children with communication problems are less likely to achieve formal qualifications at the end of compulsory schooling (Dockrell et al. 2007). According to the Bercow Review (2008), only 15 per cent of children with communication difficulties achieve five GCSE A*–C at age 16 compared to 57 per cent of all young people. So such young people may have worse employment prospects (Clegg et al. 2005).

Social impact

Again, longitudinal studies show us that children with communication difficulties early on can become adolescents with limited social participation (Tomblin 2008). In adolescence young people tend to spend less time with family and more time with peers, which is difficult for this group. They are less likely to join in conversations because they are less sensitive to others' attempts to include them, and less good at joining in themselves. This means they have fewer positive interactions. Children and young people with communication problems may be unable to communicate with others to find a resolution, discuss differences, or even share their feelings. Even if they do join in, they may experience more social stress during interactions than their peers (Wadman, Durkin and Conti-Ramsden 2011).

For some children and young people this has an impact on their ability to make and maintain friendships, particularly if they have difficulty understanding and using language to express themselves (Conti-Ramsden 2008; Fujiki et al. 2001). It is less likely to be the case if a young person is willing to help and co-operate with others. We know that friendships are very important in terms of social support and opportunities to learn about how to interact, and that isolation is a risk factor for mental health difficulties. Those without friends are at risk of loneliness and stress (Whitehouse et al. 2009a). Individuals with SEBCD are very vulnerable, not least because they are excluded from opportunities to learn about how to communicate, interact and behave appropriately if they are not able to participate socially.

Emotional and behavioural implications

It has long been recognised that communication problems are often associated with anxiety. For the child, there can be considerable frustration because they are not able to express their needs or make themselves understood. Situations where communication is difficult can generate misbehaviour. When children or young people can't understand what is expected of them or express their views, inappropriate behaviour may result. Young people with communication problems may be unable to follow routines, understand instructions, or interact appropriately at school or at home and they often receive negative attention for this, despite the fact that they don't purposely behave badly. Adolescents with communications difficulties in Tomblin's (2008) study were described as having more difficulty with compliance (following rules) than other young people, as well as compromised self-worth and self-esteem. Children with communication problems are also less likely to talk about their thoughts and feelings than their peers (Lee and Rescorla 2002).

It can be stressful for a family which has a child with communication problems. Children who have communication problems are not easy to parent because a large part of the 'management' of young children is done verbally. It is necessary for a child to understand a request in order to co-operate with it. In fact when toddlers understand adult requests, they often comply (Kaler and Kopp 1990). The reverse is also true. Parents of children with communication problems (Ollsen and Hwang 2001) also seem to be at greater risk of anxiety and depression.

Self-perception is another important factor in emotional development and it can be negatively affected in children with communication problems. For many such children, all they are aware of is failure and other people's anger and frustration. As they grow older they begin to recognise the differences between themselves and others. By the age of nine (Ackerman 1982), most children understand and can use plays on words and jokes as a means of interaction, but these are difficult to understand for children with communication problems. As their self-awareness grows, they realise that they do not have the skills to interact successfully and have fun with others. This impinges on their view of themselves (Farmer et al. 2008). Children who have poorer communication may also have lower self-esteem and are likely to have more behaviour difficulties (Durkin and Conti-Ramsden 2010).

Frustration and negative self-image may be compounded because children and young people with communication problems are more likely to be bullied than their peers (Knox and Conti-Ramsden 2007). Friendships can protect children from bullying, but as we have seen, these are difficult for some children with communication problems. The effects of bullying are obviously negative and can include anxiety and depression. Becoming a bully in response can also be a risk for those with SEBCD.

However, where children and young people with communication difficulties have good social support, when they become adults (although they may objectively have poorer skills and employment prospects), their view of their quality of life is no different than their peers' (Johnson, Beitchman and Brownlie 2010).

Children who have severe communication problems and learning difficulties which persist after they start school are at a greater risk of psychiatric difficulties as adolescents (Snowling *et al.* 2006). This includes ADHD, anxiety disorders, aggressive behaviour and even personality disorder. Adolescents who have SLI seem to have higher rates of depression and anxiety (Conti-Ramsden 2008). Conti-Ramsden (2008) found a greater risk of anxiety and depression in both male and female adolescents with SLI, whereas in the general population girls are more prone to these. However, there is no direct association between language ability and the development of mental health symptoms. The severity of communication problems does not relate to the likelihood of a mental health difficulty, but the link maybe due to a family history of communication difficulties or circumstances, such as bullying, or possibly executive function problems.

Some children with communication problems go on to develop antisocial and delinquent behaviour in the long term (Brownlie *et al.* 2004). Bryan (2004) reports how young offenders use violence when they find it difficult to communicate, are unable to make their needs known, or when they struggle to 'defend' against verbal teasing.

Gualtieri *et al.* (1983) concluded that 'disorders of the development of language are likely to be central to the development of human personality. Understanding and correcting deficiencies of language can improve behaviour and help a child resolve at least some of his emotional dilemmas' (p.169).

Potential misdiagnosis and inappropriate interventions

Children and young people who have undetected communication problems are also at risk of being misunderstood.

Cohen and Lipsett (1991) found that children who had unrecognised communication problems were 'rated by their mothers as more delinquent and by their teachers as exhibiting more psychopathology' (p.376). They concluded that it was the 'invisible' nature of some communication problems (particularly difficulty understanding language) which led people to perceive these children as more behaviourally problematic. In some cases simply the diagnosis of a communication problem improved behaviour because those talking to the child were able to accommodate their difficulties, and misunderstandings were not seen as defiance (Cohen *et al.* 1998). Some parents involved in Cohen's study reported that the assessment had helped them to understand their children's behaviour and that they had more positive interactions with them.

Perceptions of children with communication problems vary. Sometimes superficially adequate communication skills in children lead to expectations they cannot meet, and often adults use language which is far too complex. They may also be underestimated: adults sometimes view children with expressive language problems as less likeable and having less potential. If a child has difficulty interacting, his or her behaviour may be judged as 'immature', resulting in an underestimation of the child's true ability or potential. Teachers expect children to have mastered basic social skills before they start school and may project social immaturity judgements onto children with speech and language limitations (Rice, Wilcox and Hadley 1992). So these children and young people are often misunderstood; clearly this is more likely if their communication difficulties have not been recognised.

Measures of mental health and well-being sometimes require high-level language skills (Zeman *et al.* 2007), which could make it difficult for children with communication problems to express their emotional needs or concerns. Also, their emotional difficulties may be overestimated because of their poor language skills. If a differential diagnosis is based on a child's responses to questions, an inappropriate diagnosis could be reached.

Redmond and Rice (1998) investigated children with SLI and SEBD as they started school. They found that these children did not really have emotional difficulties but that their 'difficult' behaviours were just adjustments to their limited language skills. Gualtieri *et al.* (1983) argue that children with communication problems can display behaviour which could be interpreted as symptomatic of a psychiatric disorder when faced with language they cannot interpret. They may, for example, become agitated and disorganised. Children who have communication problems can seem shy and be reticent, and this can be misinterpreted as an anxiety disorder.

Another relevant factor in the misinterpretation of communication problems as behaviour difficulties is that assessments of emotional and behavioural status often have items on them which could relate to language difficulties alone rather than behaviour problems. For example, in the 'Internalizing and Attention Problem Syndrome Scales' of the Achenbach Child Behaviour Checklist (1991), there are items such as 'refuses to talk' and 'has difficulty following directions', (Redmond and Rice 1998). Therefore, according to this checklist, a child with communication problems would automatically be considered as also having behaviour difficulties.

Behaviour problems are resolved with language, and often the child's linguistic ability is overestimated. Some young children may not be able to understand conditional phrases, so the sentence 'If you do that again, X will happen' might sound like 'Do that again.' Alternatively, the consequences of their actions, couched in complex language, may not make any sense to them. Aggressive children can benefit from interventions which help to develop their understanding of social situations and social problem-solving, but how well will these interventions work if the language used to deliver them is too complex? Similarly many of the interventions for SEBD focus on aspects of language and communication, and we don't know how useful these are for those who also have communication difficulties (Im-Bolter and Cohen 2007). An example of this is that many of the interventions offered to young offenders (60 per cent or more of whom had communication difficulties) were inaccessible to them because they did not have the language skills required (Bryan *et al.* 2007).

If a young person with undetected communication difficulties is unfortunate enough to be abused or neglected which results in legal action, or if they are young offenders themselves, they can be further disadvantaged. A valid interview cannot be carried out without an understanding of the young person's language abilities. Given that many young people with communication problems have difficulty with narratives, there are major implications for their involvement in legal proceedings. Their communication difficulties should be borne in mind and questioning modified accordingly.

CASE STUDY

Anthony was 13 years old when he started at the Integrated Services Programme (ISP) school. He found it hard to learn in a group setting of five to six students, disrupting lessons with constant interruptions and persistent changes in topic. This resulted in him receiving individual tuition outside of the classroom for much of his first term. Language and communication difficulties had not been previously identified.

A speech and language therapy assessment showed that he had significant language and communication problems, including difficulty understanding what was said to him. The results of the assessment were shared with Anthony. It was suggested that one of the reasons he was getting into trouble in class, with his interruptions and changes of subject, might be because there would be less chance of misunderstanding what was being said if he wasted time or took control of the topic. This was a revelation to Anthony. He looked as if a light bulb had just been switched on in his head. 'So that's what's wrong with me!' he exclaimed.

Over the next few weeks, Anthony was back in class for the majority of his lesson, and there was a significant reduction in his interruptions and disruptive behaviours. What was startling about this dramatic turn-around was that he had barely started speech and language therapy. The changes in his behaviour appeared to relate to just knowing that he had language and communication problems. His unidentified language difficulties had exacerbated existing behaviour and educational problems.

Conclusion and implications

Difficulties in identifying communication problems and indeed in defining them affect estimates of prevalence and public perception.

However, communication problems have far-reaching negative implications, so a speech and language assessment should be a routine part of the management of children with SEBD. This is particularly important, as there is also some evidence of a worsening of language difficulties if they remain unsuspected, and for some, improvement if they are identified (Cohen *et al.* 1998).

In Steer's review of behavioural issues in school, it is stressed that 'Consideration should always be given to whether a child's behavioural difficulties arise from an underlying learning difficulty that has not been identified, or is not being appropriately addressed' (Steer 2009, point 56).

There is also a need for increased awareness of language development and impairment amongst professionals working with children with SEBD, so that they can accommodate children's communication problems. If children have SEBCD, it is essential to understand their language capabilities in order to help them resolve other difficulties.

Communication skills are a protective factor against mental health difficulties (DCSF 2008b) as well as being a key life skill, so unaddressed communication difficulties in those who have SEBD are also a public health issue.

Chapter 4

Language and Social Disadvantage

Communication Difficulties in Vulnerable Children and Young People

Language and social disadvantage

There is accumulating evidence that children and young people from areas of social disadvantage often have the additional challenge of communication problems. As we have seen, communication problems can bring with them many risks, and for vulnerable children and young people these can further restrict life chances and increase the likelihood of social exclusion. Children and young people in areas of social deprivation are also more likely to have behavioural issues (Washbrook 2010).

> Social exclusion is a complex and multi-dimensional process. It involves the lack or denial of resources, rights, goods and services, and the inability to participate in the normal relationships and activities available to the majority of people in a society, whether in economic, social, cultural or political arenas. It affects both the quality of life of individuals and the equity and cohesion of society as a whole. (Levitas *et al.* 2007, p.9)

Poverty of communication skills in children with low SES is identifiable early on, even at 14 months (Rowe and Goldin-Meadow 2009). There are also differences in the size of vocabulary between children with low and high SES from an early age (Hart and Risley 1995); this gap widens until age four then remains relatively constant (Farkas and Beron 2004; Waldfogel 2010). There are also other differences in communication skills which persist. In the UK, a group of 240 children in an area of social deprivation had their language skills assessed as they entered school; over half of them had delayed language development, and this was still the case two years later, although they had no learning difficulties (Locke and Ginsborg 2003). What was most concerning in this study was that some children's communication skills deteriorated. Socio-economic status also affects access to services: over half of the children identified as having communication difficulties in one study had not been referred to speech and language therapy, and these children had lower socio-economic backgrounds than children who had been referred (Bishop and McDonald 2009).

In secondary schools in areas of social disadvantage, there is a similar pattern of many pupils having limited language skills, which are often unrecognised, and SEBD (Stringer 2006). Indeed, low SES is a risk factor for developing communication difficulties and social, emotional and behavioural difficulties (Roseberry-McKibbin 2007) as well as mental health difficulties (Emerson and Hatton 2007). For example, the effects of maternal depression on the language development of children seems to be more severe in mothers of low SES (Stein *et al.* 2008).

It can be argued that these language or communication differences are differences in register, style or code, but the fact remains that many children do not have the appropriate communication skills for the settings they find themselves in – for example school and sometimes, unfortunately, the legal system. As Feinstein, Duckworth and Sabates (2004, p.22) say, 'Language pervades the transmission of human and cultural capital from birth', so those whose communication skills are limited are especially at risk of disadvantage and further social exclusion. Young people with undetected communication problems recognise that they may not know 'big words', and express frustration at not being able to explain things and at not being able to understand teachers. They are also unfamiliar with the idea of getting help to develop their communication skills (Spencer *et al.* 2010), which is both feasible and effective.

Groups which are at risk of social exclusion are also at risk of undetected communication difficulties: adolescents in areas of social disadvantage (Myers and Botting 2008), children with SEBD, those excluded from school, looked-after children and young offenders.

Why is there a link between language and social advantage?
Language input

Language levels at entry to preschool seem to be important in the link between SES and educational achievement, and therefore much of the effect of SES impacts when children are very young (Durham *et al.* 2007). Rowe and Goldin-Meadow (2009) found that differences in children's vocabulary at 54 months correlated with gesture use by these children at 14 months, which in turn correlated to the amount of gesture their parents used to them when they were young. So those whose parents gestured more had a larger vocabulary at 54 months – and these were children from more privileged backgrounds. Children in families with high SES also hear language which is more varied in terms of vocabulary and more complicated in its structure; this then relates to the children's vocabulary skills (Huttenlocher *et al.* 2007). It is important to note that children with low SES may have fewer words, but they do not seem to have a difficulty learning new words (Horton-Ikard and Weismer 2007), so in this respect they may be different from other children with communication problems.

However, as we have seen in Chapter 1, the key factor in helping children's language develop is positive responsive interactions: not just talking to or at them, but listening and showing an interest in what they want to say. Narrative skills are important, and it seems to help children develop these skills when adults focus on the child's topic of interest and ask them to elaborate (Peterson and Roberts 2003). It is important to remember that just because language input relates to SES, it doesn't mean that parental input is cause rather than effect. In a responsive interaction, adults respond to the language levels and abilities of the child.

Parenting style

There seem to be differences in how much parents actively teach their children language, reasoning and negotiation skills (Lareau 2003), and the amount of parental support children get in school is influential in their progress (Desforges and Abouchaar 2003). Activities such as reading with children and creating opportunities to play with other children lead to better outcomes (Sammons *et al.* 2002). Parental style of interaction also affects a child's ability to learn. In Hart and Risley's (1995) work, middle-class children were five times as likely to get positive feedback as children on welfare, and the lower SES children were twice as likely to be told 'no'; but of course some children are easier to parent than others, and it is difficult to tell whether parental style is cause or effect. However, an effort to 'teach' some parents, perhaps persuaded by toy manufacturers, may underestimate the value of positive interactions and free play (Hirsch-Pacek and Michnick Golinkoff 2003).

A communication legacy

Parents who did not finish secondary school are at risk of having children with communication difficulties (Campbell *et al.* 2003), perhaps because they are unsure how to help language develop (Torr 2004). It is difficult to help your child to develop skills that you don't have or give them experiences you didn't have. It's also important to remember the genetic and other environmental influences in language development. Children from disadvantaged backgrounds take longer to develop their theory of mind than children from middle-class backgrounds, perhaps because of differences in 'mind mindedness', which is more prevalent in middle-class interactions (Hughes *et al.* 2005).

Environmental factors

The negative impact of poverty on all areas of a child's development must never be underestimated. Some families are under multiple stresses that make it difficult for them to be responsive to their children in ways that can help language develop (Pickstone 2006). Family income is the best predictor of a child's communication skills, and parents of disabled children are at risk of poverty (Sharma 2007). Factors which seem to help reduce the effects of early language problems are the child being born into an employed family, parental education beyond minimum school-leaving age, good housing, and going to preschool (Schoon *et al.* 2010).

Vulnerable groups with an increased risk of communication problems

Children who have been abused and neglected

Children who have been abused and neglected are very likely to have impaired emotional, language and cognitive development (Fonagy, Gergely and Target 2007). Abused and neglected children are less likely to play symbolically or with other children; they may show less empathy and find it difficult to calm down or otherwise regulate their behaviour. Toddlers who have been maltreated are much less likely to have language for internal states: thoughts and feelings (Beeghly and Cicchetti 1994). Their delay in emotional development also shows in difficulties recognising facial expressions. Fonagy *et al.* (2007) argue that in abusive relationships, open, reflective communication about how the child feels is, almost by definition, compromised. Therefore such children and young people often have difficulties with communication.

Children who have been abused or neglected have greater needs for medical and special educational services than other children. In a survey of over 5000 abused and neglected children in the US, more than a third had special health needs, and the risk was greater if they were fostered or adopted (Ringeisen *et al.* 2008). This is likely to include needs for services to help develop their communication skills. One study (Noll *et al.* 2010) followed girls who had been sexually abused as children for 18 years: their ability to understand language developed at a slower rate and they reached a lower level of proficiency than their non-abused peers. Their educational attainment was also significantly affected.

Having communication difficulties may even increase the risk of being abused. One study found that women with communication problems had a history of more abusive experiences than controls (Brownlie *et al.* 2007). There is a strong link between childhood abuse and neglect and stressors on the family (Herrenkohl and Herrenkohl 2007), underlining the importance of considering multiple risk factors in cases of abuse and neglect, including language and social exclusion.

Children in public care

Children in public care are also known as 'looked-after children', 'children in statutory care', 'children in non-maternal care' and 'children in the care of the local authority'. Children come into 'care' either voluntarily or where social services can show that the child or young person is suffering, or is likely to suffer 'significant harm' if left in the parents' care, either because the level of care is inadequate or because he or she is beyond parental control. In 2009, about 56,000 children were in statutory care in the UK. These children have often been affected by parental substance abuse, abuse or neglect, domestic violence, poor housing or frequent moves, poverty, or homelessness, and they may also have special needs or disabilities. They often come from families with few resources or little support. Children in public care are more likely to have educational, psychiatric and neuro-developmental difficulties than even the most deprived children living at home (Ford *et al.* 2007). About 80 per cent of looked-after children have behavioural problems (Leslie *et al.* 2005), which may be related to the fact that looked-after children are eight times as likely to be excluded from school as other children (Ofsted 2008a). What is disappointing is that, although there has been progress, they still do not always have their additional needs recognised and met.

The educational attainment of children in public care is lower than for other groups. In 2008, 14 per cent of children in public care achieved five A*–C grades at the end of statutory schooling, compared to 65.3 per cent for all children. The educational needs of children in public care may not be recognised; there might be unreasonably low expectations of them, or their special needs may not be recognised. Some suggest that socio-economic risk factors are what lead to poor educational outcomes rather than being in care per se (Berridge 2007).

Sixty per cent of those going into public care have mental health difficulties (Meltzer *et al.* 2003), in comparison to one in ten in the typical population. Those in public care still have poorer access to mental health services (Mooney *et al.* 2009), and there may be difficulties in sharing information and inadequate assessment. In the Ofsted (2010a) report on the provision of mental health services for looked-after children, there is hardly any mention of communication difficulties except to say that if such problems were present advocates would be used – but clearly this can only happen if communication difficulties have been adequately identified.

The common assessment framework (part of a system which aims to achieve multi-professional support for the most vulnerable children) in England and Wales does contain a section on speech, language and communication, but it remains to be seen how effective this assessment is at identifying previously undetected communication problems. It is a step forwards in developing multi-agency assessment and information-sharing for vulnerable children and young people, but it is time consuming and therefore often only available where resources allow (Gilligan and Mamby 2008). The implementation of a screening for developmental difficulties in young children in foster care in the US doubled the detection of such difficulties (Jee *et al.* 2010), which implies that current systems for identifying needs are inadequate. The greatest barrier to meeting these children's needs is their frequent changes of placement and of the professionals working with them. Children and young people in public care stress the negative effects of discontinuity and want more choice in the sorts of support they receive (Stanley 2007).

In the context of such unmet needs, it is not startling that communication problems in children in public care also go undetected. The rate of identified communication difficulties in looked-after children is twice as prevalent as in the typical population, at 16 per cent (Meltzer *et al.* 2003). There is also some evidence of a much greater number of undetected communication problems in looked-after children (Cross 1999, 2001). However, non-maternal care in the first year of life can help develop a child's communication skills, especially if they are from a low SES background (Geoffroy *et al.* 2007).

Children excluded from school

Children and young people are excluded from school when their behaviour is unacceptable. Children from lower socio-economic groups are eight times as likely to have behaviour problems as those from wealthier backgrounds (Propper and Rigg 2007). This is in the context of children with SEBD being disadvantaged, in that they were the least likely to receive effective support and the most likely to receive support too late (Ofsted 2006). Those excluded from school are likely to be disadvantaged in some way. Although exclusion may make it easier for those who remain to teach and learn, there are no clear advantages to the young people themselves. Children most likely to be excluded from school are those in public care, those from areas of social deprivation, children with SEBD and, amongst other factors, boys (Achilles, Mclaughlin and Croninger 2007). The other group at risk of exclusion is those who have SEN. The Lamb enquiry (DSCF 2009) stated that it was not acceptable for children with SEN to be eight times as likely as other pupils to be excluded from school. Amongst those at risk of exclusion from school are children and young people who have undetected communication problems. In an area of socio-economic deprivation, a preliminary study found that 10 of 15 teenage pupils at risk of exclusion from school had previously unrecognised communication difficulties (Clegg *et al.* 2009).

Clearly children and young people who are vulnerable do not necessarily thrive in mainstream schools. Perhaps their needs and ways of learning can't be accommodated there. Pupils themselves may have difficulty accepting other pupils who have SEBD (Visser and Dubsky 2009) as well as those with communication difficulties. A recent review of the literature found that there is little evidence overall of any positive effects of including children with SEN in mainstream schools (Lindsay 2007). Key factors for good progress for children with SEN in mainstream schools seem to be 'the involvement of a specialist teacher; good assessment; work tailored to challenge pupils sufficiently; and commitment from school leaders to ensure good progress for all pupils' (Ofsted 2006, p.2). However, if children with SEBCD can't be educated in the mainstream, are they offered adequate alternatives? Do schools for children with SEBD understand and address the potential communication difficulties of these pupils, in a routine and evidence-based way? The evidence for undetected communication problems in these settings suggests not.

Not in education, employment or training (NEETs)

Many of those excluded from schools are at risk of not being employed or in training or education (NEET). The most successful services offered to such young people offer help to resolve personal and social problems as well as offering co-ordinated multi-professional services. Where school has not been a positive experience, short, flexible courses matched to the needs and interests of young people are often more successful. There is emerging evidence that this group is also at increased risk of communication problems (Elliott in preparation). Good communication skills are increasingly prized by employers, and young people without them are at a distinct disadvantage.

Young offenders

Sadly, the vulnerable young people previously considered in this section are all at greater risk of becoming young offenders. Many young offenders have experienced harsh parenting, neglect or abuse (Bowlby 1969). It's a well-worn 'career' path that a greater focus on developing communication skills could help dismantle. As we have seen, young offenders are also at considerable risk of having undetected and unaddressed communication difficulties (Bryan et al. 2007). Current systems do not record additional learning needs accurately (Ofsted 2010b), and the young people themselves describe the difficulties they experience with listening, thinking, speaking and reading (Sanger et al. 2003). The difficulties they have with telling their story so that others can understand (Snow and Powell 2005) have far-reaching implications in terms of them getting into trouble and getting out of it. In one study, young people who were deemed responsible for a delinquent act had poorer language skills, and the majority of these had not been previously identified as having difficulties with language (Blanton and Dagenais 2007). Were they actually responsible, or were they unable to explain their situation? There is also evidence of limited vocabulary in this group, and concerns that they may not be able to access verbally mediated interventions which are aimed at their rehabilitation (Bryan *et al.* 2007).

Conclusion and implications

Undetected communication problems in vulnerable groups is a serious and ongoing problem. Limited communication skills are likely to contribute to further social exclusion in addition to the other risks associated with communication difficulties. Vocabulary at age five is the best predictor of whether children who experienced social deprivation could 'buck the trend' and escape poverty in later life (Blanden 2006), and these are skills we know how to teach.

There are also serious additional risks for vulnerable groups of children and young people linked to their communication problems. Children's credibility, whether they are victims of abuse or young offenders, is often based on the quality of their narratives (Newman and McGregor 2006), and of course the credibility of the young person will affect the decisions made about them. It must be stressed here that a child's ability to construct a coherent narrative is not related to the facts of the matter, what actually happened or their role in it. It is important therefore for everyone working with vulnerable groups to be aware of their potential communication difficulties. Training may be necessary both to recognise the child or young person's communication problems and to modify one's own language accordingly. For example, using open-ended questions is most effective to elicit the best quality story from a child or young person who may have been abused (Feltis *et al.* 2010).

I have heard people say, 'This sort of limited communication is just typical of children in this area, and we can't do anything about it', but this thinking needs to be challenged. It probably is true that communication difficulties and social disadvantage are linked, but that doesn't mean that nothing could or should be done about it. As Hart and Risley's (1995) work showed, responsive interactions (not just exposure to language), encouragement, interest in children's thoughts and feelings, and positive emotions rather than stress seemed to stimulate verbal and other abilities.

Chapter 5

The Identification and Assessment of Communication Difficulties in Children with SEBD

Introduction

In this chapter there is a discussion about types of communication problems as well as the merits of various methods of identifying and assessing them. Given the negative effects of communication difficulties and their often 'invisible' nature, their identification and assessment is important. In 1996, Beitchman and Cohen established that children who had communication problems identified at age five were likely to have poorer linguistic and academic outcomes at age 12 than their peers. They concluded that 'These findings reveal the urgent need for early intervention among children with pervasive speech/language impairment' (p.804). Their sentiments have been echoed by many since, but this hasn't necessarily translated into practice, especially for children with SEBCD. The first step towards this is accurate and early identification of communication problems.

Obviously, effective support (including teaching communication skills, adult modifications of interactions, adaptations of the tasks and the environment) can only occur if communication problems are recognised. Behaviours may be interpreted differently once the adults realise a child or young person has communication problems. When adults understand children's linguistic limitations, they can see them in a more positive light, enabling a better assessment of behavioural difficulties. Parents, who have a better understanding of their child's communication problems, are less likely to be influenced by their children's communication problems when rating their behaviour (Lindsay et al. 2007).

However, there is no consensus about how best to detect communication problems; many options are available. The type of assessment used will be influenced by the reason for carrying out the assessment. Assessment may take place for research purposes, but mostly it occurs in order to identify those eligible for services and to guide interventions and measure progress. Some kinds of assessment may be useful for identification per se, but other forms of assessment may provide more useful descriptive information for developing teaching and therapy plans and measuring outcomes.

Law and Conway (1989) suggest that an ongoing assessment of the communication skills of children in public care might be a 'barometer' of the success of the placement. No child psychiatric assessment is complete without a developmental assessment, which should include communication skills, as this not only has a bearing on behaviour but also on the effectiveness of any intervention.

When an assessment is requested, it is important to be clear about the following:

- What information is needed and by whom? Will it just confirm what is already known?

- Who will it benefit? Is this for adults, or the child or young person?

- Is the aim to compare the child or young person's communication skills to a cross-section of the population?

- Is this about access to services?

- Is it most useful to assess the child or young person or the communicative environment?

What are communication problems and how are they identified?

There is no simple answer to this because 'adequate communication' is hard to define. Language itself is a moving target; it is continually changing and being added to, especially by teenagers. Language also varies greatly according to the socio-economic, minority and educational status of those using it. Individuals also vary the language they use according to where they are and who they are talking to. Consequently, identifying communication problems is not straightforward; it is both difficult to identify 'norms' and to judge how effectively someone varies their communication across settings and with different people.

Labels, definitions or descriptions?

One of the key issues in assessment is its purpose. One reason for doing an assessment might be to assign the appropriate label or diagnosis. As noted previously, a wide range of loosely defined terms are used to describe communication problems. The technical use of everyday words such as 'speech', 'language' and 'communication', probably adds to the confusion that exists in identifying or even discussing communication problems. There are yet another set of *formal* definitions or diagnoses.

Formal diagnoses are provided in the International Classification of Diseases (World Health Organization 2007), which has the following categories:

- specific speech articulation disorder
- expressive language disorder
- receptive language disorder
- acquired aphasia with epilepsy, known as Landau-Kleffner syndrome
- other developmental disorder of speech and language, unspecified.

The Diagnostic and Statistical Manual of Mental Disorders, also known as the DSM-IV, published by the American Psychiatric Association (1994) lists:

- expressive language disorder
- mixed receptive-expressive language disorder
- phonological disorder
- stuttering
- communication disorder not otherwise specified.

What these have in common is a very broad view of the types of communication difficulties, such as whether they are to do with understanding or expressing oneself or with speech sounds. The fact that they differ is interesting, but more importantly, they omit difficulties with the use of language, although these can exist separately from ASD (Bishop and Norbury 2002). These categorisations are important because they can be helpful in research and in identifying whether groups have different outcomes or respond differently to intervention. However, they are not necessarily helpful in practice, because they don't provide enough detail to guide intervention or give any information on the practical or functional effects of these difficulties.

An important diagnosis which is used in practice as well as in research is SLI. This is where language skills are said to be particularly impaired in relation to non-verbal intelligence (NVIQ); 7 per cent of all children have SLI (Tomblin et al. 1997). However, there are difficulties using NVIQ as a reference because children may get low scores for reasons other than limited intelligence, for example anxiety, unfamiliarity or, indeed, limited language. Another problem with this type of discrepancy criteria is that it is difficult to assess non-verbal skills (Bishop 1994). Even tests of NVIQ require the use of language skills (Lahey 1990), so children with language deficits may fail on these tasks, too. Children with SLI also have non-verbal difficulties, for example with visual processing, so this further confounds the distinction.

The category of SLI is not used for children with SEBD, as it is said to exist in the absence of any other developmental difficulties. However, as research has continued it has become more obvious that although those with SLI do seem to have particular problems with language, they often have other difficulties too, including SEBDs. It may also be the case that SLI is not as distinct from other developmental disorders as was once thought. There are overlaps between SLI and dyslexia (Catts et al. 2005) as well as speech sound disorders in children (Pennington and Bishop 2009). SLI and ADHD (McGrath et al. 2008) often seem to occur together, and SLI and ASD may be less distinct than we thought (Tager-Flusberg 2006), as some children show the characteristics of both.

The key question is whether NVIQ affects progress in intervention. This argument about 'potential' is often used in the allocation of speech and language therapy services or for entry into special units for children with SLI. However, NVIQ does not necessarily help predict who will benefit from language intervention (Tomblin, Records and Zhang 1996). In practice, the outcomes for children with poor language skills, whether their non-verbal ability is moderately limited or within the typical range, are similar (Tomblin 2008) and tend not to be positive. Some researchers would suggest that all children with communication problems should receive services to help develop their language skills, regardless of any additional moderate learning difficulties (Rice et al. 2004) because progress is similar in both groups (Fey, Long and Cleave 1994).

In considering labels or diagnoses, it is important to be aware of the possibility of developmental disorders occurring together: children with learning difficulties, ASD, ADHD, dyspraxia and dyslexia and, of course, SEBD are likely to have communication problems as well. However, the idea of excluding other possible causes of communication problems is a useful one, as it can guide intervention. When assessing children with SEBD for communication problems, it is important to rule out factors like attention deficits, which can appear to be comprehension difficulties. Children with ADHD have difficulty following instructions and listening, and it is not always easy to determine whether this is due to comprehension difficulties or attention problems. However, if their inattention is more marked during verbal tasks, it is reasonable to assume that a communication difficulty is a contributory factor. ADHD alone is more likely to be the cause if inattention is also present during tasks with fewer verbal demands (Prizant *et al.* 1990).

If a communication problem exists where a child's or young person's skills are significantly below expectations for children of that developmental level, then 'significantly below' must be defined. In terms of identifying when language development is unusual, how far behind one's peers does a child have to be? There is considerable variation in the rate at which all children acquire language, so it is not always clear where atypical development is occurring. Although many children who begin to talk later than others go on to have communication problems, not all of them do (Rice, Taylor and Zubrick 2008). It is not always the case that children and young people with communication problems get low scores on assessments, either; they may even score within the expected range (Spaulding, Plante and Farinella 2006). A decision has to be made whether a communication difficulty is defined by a statistically unusual score or by its negative effects on everyday interactions.

Funding can also be relevant here: if there is only funding for the lowest two per cent of the population to receive help (as in some parts of the US), only this portion of the population will be defined as communication-impaired. Special education provision for children with communication problems may be limited to those that are seen to have the most severe problems in the absence of other learning difficulties, despite the limitations of this approach.

Perhaps the most useful definition for identifying communication problems is in terms of the practical effects of these difficulties for the person experiencing them. Can a young person use language to interact well with peers, make friends and access the curriculum? Communication problems identified by any other means, without reference to their practical consequences, may not really exist as problems for the child or young person who experiences them. Indeed, the young person concerned or their caregivers may be the best judges of whether or not they are experiencing problems with communication, although they may not be able to explain or define them. Furthermore, communication problems can probably best be defined when they lead to an unacceptable risk for undesirable outcomes (Tomblin 2008).

In order to develop an intervention programme, a detailed description of the communication problems a child or young person experiences and their functional effects is most useful. Then it will be necessary to measure progress, which might require a different type of assessment.

Which language skills should be assessed in children with SEBD?

Before identifying an assessment tool, it is necessary to decide which communication skills should be assessed. There is a large range of assessments to choose from, none of which assess all communication skills. So decisions have to be made about where to start with an assessment and, indeed, when to stop. The choice of assessment will obviously be influenced by its aim, but are there areas of communication which are likely to be particularly difficult for children with SEBD? The answers found by research depend on the assessments used in that research, the research design and particularly the size of the study sample. Often the information available is from small-scale studies of slightly different populations, so it's difficult to draw any broad conclusions. However, we know that the links between SEBD and communication problems are weakest if the child in question has difficulty with speech sounds, so this is not necessarily an area to focus on. Such communication problems are the hardest to miss!

The social 'use' of language has long been identified as a particular area of difficulty in children with SEBD (McDonough 1989). These young people have difficulty with skills such as giving an appropriate amount of information, appreciating another person's point of view and being aware of how context influences communication. Not only is there a high correlation between difficulties with the use of language and SEBD, but it is also suggested that an early assessment of the social use of language could identify underlying difficulties such as ADHD and ASD (Ketelaars *et al.* 2010). It is important to reiterate that difficulties with the use of language can occur in the absence of ASD (Bishop and Norbury 2002). Therefore, an assessment of social communication skills or the way children 'use' language is an important part of any assessment of a young person with SEBCD. Commonly used assessments of this area are the Children's Communication Checklist, or CCC, (Bishop 1998) and, in Canada, the Language Use Inventory (O'Neill 2007).

Beyond the likelihood of problems with the use of language, it is not clear which other communication problems are most likely. One study in schools found that expressive language difficulties were most common in students with SEBD (Nelson, Benner and Cheney 2005), and another found that mixed receptive expressive difficulties were most common (Clegg *et al.* 2009). It may be the case that problems with the form of language alone are not associated with SEBD (Mackie and Law 2010), but further research is necessary.

Narrative skills are often particularly problematic for young people with SEBD. The narrative skills of young offenders were found to be significantly worse than those of comparable young people (Snow and Powell 2005). To tell a story, one needs not only mastery of the structure of language, its grammar and vocabulary, but also to be able to coherently sequence events, take the viewpoint of the characters and appreciate the listener's knowledge and perspective. Narratives are also important for self-concept. We develop our own self-concept through stories about our experiences and the stories we share with others; most of our interactions are laced with anecdotes. We also need narratives to explain what happened and get ourselves out of trouble. Oral narrative skills are a predictor of success with literacy. Many communication and emotional skills contribute to a coherent meaningful narrative, so it's an important skill to assess in this population. They can be assessed using the Expression, Reception and Recall of Narrative Instrument, or ERRNI (Bishop 2004), or the Assessment of Comprehension and Expression (Adams *et al.* 2001).

Another area of difficulty for many children and young people with SEBD is emotion vocabulary. The ability to name emotions is a predictor of successful social interaction (Miller *et al.* 2005), so a baseline of these skills is useful in order to measure progress.

It must be stressed that any area of language could be impaired, so although we have some clues as to what to assess, it is important to assess form, content and use. It is also vital to remember the particularly invisible nature of comprehension problems and the negative consequences associated with them.

A holistic approach

The holistic approach to assessment stresses the inter-relatedness of language, thinking and emotions, and it is increasingly used in the identification and treatment of communication problems. The holistic approach considers the young person's communicative strengths and weaknesses and their effects, as well as the context in which these occur. It also tries to understand the young person's overall development, his or her family and community situation and sense of self and social effectiveness. The World Health Organization's International Classification of Functioning (ICF) is an example of a holistic framework which can be used to guide assessment. It aims to provide a view of disability from a biological, individual and social perspective.

In this framework, *disability* includes:

- impairments, e.g. difficulties with interpreting speech sounds, which can lead to activity limitations

- activity limitations, e.g. problems understanding what others say, which can result in participation restrictions

- participation restrictions, e.g. hampering social interaction or by limiting their access to lessons.

This sort of model makes it clear how some people are 'disabled' by the environment they find themselves in as well as the difficulties they may have with communication.

The holistic approach assumes that an assessment of communication skills is part of an assessment of the young person's overall functioning, but of course this is not always the case. Nonetheless, it is important to gather information about other areas of functioning apart from communication, particularly if the young person appears to have complex needs. Developmental history, school performance, family history, temperament and environmental and cultural factors could all be relevant. A hearing screening is always necessary when communication problems are suspected. Information about cognitive and emotional skills can be useful. An assessor must also be aware of the typical stages of child development, for example in levels of attention and typical emotional development as well as language development. As part of a communication assessment it is clearly very important to find out which languages children and young people are exposed to and speak.

Gathering information from people who know the child or young person well, as well as from the young person him- or herself, also contributes to a holistic view of communication skills and problems. It is important for the interviewer to collaborate with these 'significant others' and enable them to take an active part in the assessment process. Good collaboration during the assessment process can be therapeutic in itself, because a greater understanding of the communication problems a young person faces enables better planning and intervention.

Law and Conway (1989) suggest that a thorough assessment of communication skills is particularly important in children with SEBD, as focusing on one area and neglecting any other can result in a misleading picture. The precise nature of the assessment will depend on the child's age and abilities. The 'use' of language for preverbal children will be mainly vocalisations and gestures and may also include signs or symbols. It is important to determine which communicative functions are being expressed. Sometimes children will use unusual or unacceptable ways of communicating, and these should be recognised and analysed as a first step towards helping the development of more acceptable forms of communication (Wetherby and Prizant 1992).

No single assessment can evaluate the complex interplays between language, cognition and emotion, so a holistic approach will usually include a mixture of formal (where the process is strictly defined) and informal (more flexible in their delivery) assessments as well as observation in different contexts and interviewing significant others. A combination of parental reports and standardised tests seem to be the most effective way of identifying communication difficulties (Bishop and McDonald 2009). A triangulation of data gathered in different ways will help to build up an accurate picture of any communication difficulties. For example, comprehension can be assessed in context (How does a child respond to an instruction in class?). It can also be assessed in a de-contextualised situation by formal testing, and people who know the child well can provide information about functional effects of comprehension problems (refusal to work, irritation where adults use complex language, etc.). If several methods indicate problems in an area, it is more likely that this is a significant issue for the young person. Expressive language assessment needs to occur in different ways too. The nature of the task, as well as the context and the conversational partner, will influence the complexity of the language the young person uses, so the use of a variety of assessments will lead to a truer picture. It is also important to take notice of behaviours and strategy use during assessment, which can give insight into attention, response times, motivation and problem-solving skills, all of which are important for helping the child or young person move forward.

Assessing the communication skills of children and young people with SEBD

Young people who have SEBD have them for a reason. Knowledge of their family background, as well as their developmental, emotional and medical history, are crucial to understanding and helping them feel able to take part in an assessment. However, as well as knowing as much as is possible about a young person, an open mind is also necessary. Often children and young people with SEBD have a considerable negative reputation, but it is important to have positive expectations of them because these can be a self-fulfilling prophecy. Day-to-day information is also important during an assessment as events in the young person's life, such as a parent leaving home, a pending court case, a change of placement or the teacher being on a course, can markedly affect how the child responds.

Consent for an assessment has to be gained from whoever has parental responsibility and, of course, the young person himself or herself. Confidentiality is also an issue here, and it is important to be clear about whom the assessment is for and who will have access to it. The young person involved needs a clear explanation of the purpose of the assessment, including the possible outcomes and implications. Often, a good place to start is finding out what the child or young person thinks of their communication skills, perhaps using a checklist like the communication checklist to self-report (Bishop, Whitehouse and Sharpe 2009). Does this assessment fit in with the young person's concerns and goals (see Spencer, Clegg and Stackhouse 2010)? Clearly, all of this has to be carefully and sensitively done, but honesty is important, as it is an integral part of the process of gaining trust and co-operation. Co-operation can be encouraged, depending on the child's age, either through intrinsic rewards, such as 'This will help me help you to understand what your teacher says', or extrinsic rewards, like 'Let's do this and then you can choose something to play with for five minutes'. The best, but most time-consuming, approach is to give the child or young person time to get to know the person assessing them, listen and value their experiences and build rapport.

The environment in which the assessment takes place will have an impact on the results. A clinical setting is anxiety-provoking for most people; therefore it is important that assessments are carried out in a variety of situations. Young children will be more relaxed, but possibly more distracted, at home. A school-aged child might find it easier to complete formal assessment if they have already met the assessor, perhaps when the assessor came to observe them in class. The assessor needs to be aware of whether a pupil is happy to come out of class or whether they would see this as an unbearable stigma. Likewise, what are the effects of an unfamiliar adult observing them in class or at play? Ideally, a room for formal testing should not be intimidating but a quiet, comfortable place free of distractions.

Being assessed is emotionally charged. It is best to acknowledge this and be very sensitive to how the young person is feeling. They need time to get to know and trust the assessor and to feel safe. They should be encouraged to say how they feel, and to say when they are tired or when they need to let off steam. From the children's or young people's point of view, they are trying to work out what they should do or say in a strange situation, where they are unsure of the social rules and may feel powerless. Planning and flexibility are both important; the assessor must be willing to negotiate about the order of events, and how much 'work' the young person does. Young people with SEBD may be anxious, eager to please, unco-operative or passive. (There is never a dull moment.) They may have short attention spans and be distractible, so it is wise to a have a variety of activities available so that ones which are motivating, and at the right level of difficulty, can be used. The impulsivity of children with ADHD will affect their performance on assessments, so alertness to how they respond as well as to what their responses are is necessary.

Being responsive to young people being assessed is necessary because it is often impossible to predict how they'll be feeling and what they'll be happy to do. Children with SEBD can become non-compliant or oppositional when the demands of the task are beyond them, or when they do not understand what to do. If this happens, it's important to have a change of activity available and acknowledge 'I didn't explain that very well' or 'That doesn't make any sense, does it? Let's do something else'. If young people have a short attention span, frequent changes of activity and 'rest periods' will help them focus for longer. For some children, an unstructured 'free play' situation is extremely anxiety-producing, while others find it relaxing. Some respond well to being given clear choices, though others will find this stressful. Many children prefer structure and a clear list of 'jobs' to be done during the session, but others will find this daunting. It may be necessary to modify assessments, because they often can't all be completed in one attempt, but careful note should be taken of how and why modifications are done, as this provides useful information and it may also affect the way the results are interpreted. The children's or young people's views on their performance also provide valuable insights. Unco-operativeness is often cited as a reason why a child or young person could not be assessed. However, what can't be assessed is as important as what can; these are all useful clues. Information gathered from others and observations are particularly important if a young person is not keen to undertake formal assessment.

A holistic approach is extremely important with young people who have SEBD. Involving the family where possible and other people who know the child well will help determine whether their behaviour and responses in the assessment process are representative. If the results from different assessments concur, they are easier to interpret – although of course the opposite is also true! It is likely that assessing the communication skills of a young person with SEBD will be very time-consuming.

Screening/clinical markers

Is there a simple way of identifying children who may have communication difficulties, a way which could possibly be carried out by non-experts, thereby identifying who should go on to have a fuller assessment? A screening test should be able to pick out which children are at risk from long-term or serious communication problems without missing any and without identifying children to be at risk when they are not (false positives). One risk with a simple screening is that if you just look at one area, for example vocabulary, you may well miss gaps in other communication skills. In order to devise a screening test, it is necessary to know what are the early signs or basis of communication problems, sometimes called 'clinical markers'.

In some children with communication problems, difficulty with processing speech sounds is present from an early age (Weber *et al.* 2005). Such auditory information processing is critical for language development, and children with SLI have difficulties with sentence repetition tasks which rely on this skill (Devescovi and Caselli 2007). Tests of auditory information processing such as non-word repetition or sentence repetition are useful because they are not reliant on previous knowledge, language or context. An example of this kind of assessment is asking a child to repeat a non-word, for example 'tep'; only those with an intact sound-processing capacity will find this sort of task easy. Young children with communication problems were seven times more likely to have difficulty with a non-word repetition task as typically developing children (Chiat and Roy 2008). Non-word repetition also correlates to vocabulary size, at least in two-year-olds (Stokes and Klee 2009). Giddan *et al.* (1996) found a high proportion of children with previously unsuspected communication problems and SEBD had similar auditory processing difficulties.

Another possible 'basis' of communication difficulties is limitations in early social communication skills, such as joint attention. The idea is not that these are all that is necessary for the appropriate development of the 'use' of language, but their absence might point to underlying difficulties in this area. In Chiat and Roy's 2008 study, the most significant early predictor of persisting communication problems was difficulty with understanding language, although word repetition skills predicted later grammatical ability, and early social communication skills predicted later ones. So there is unlikely to be just one clinical marker or early sign of later communication problems, but we are learning more about what the significant factors could be.

Another approach is to try to identify risk factors in the child's history which put him or her at risk of communication problems. Generally such screening has proved ineffective so far because we don't know enough about what to look for. The US Department of Health carried out a review of the evidence for screening in 2006 and concluded that the 'use of risk factors to guide selective screening is not supported by studies' (p.6). A recent study (Reilly *et al.* 2009) looked at the following: gender, preterm birth, birth weight, multiple birth, birth order, SES, maternal mental health, maternal vocabulary and education, maternal age at birth of child, non-English-speaking background, and a family history of speech and/or language difficulties, and found that these were unlikely to be helpful in predicting language delay.

It might be useful to bolster a screening by using other sources of information and assessment. There is some evidence that parental report measures can identify children with communication problems (Skarakis, Campbell and Dempsey 2009). Also Pickstone (2003) found that workers without a professional training were able to carry out an effective screening for children with language delay as part of a Sure Start (Glass 2001) initiative. However, previously, screening using both a structured test or a parent-led model has been found to be ineffective in that many children with communication problems were not identified and some whose language was developing typically were identified as having communication problems (Laing *et al.* 2002). Nonetheless, there are continued attempts to design a useful screen, some using clinical markers, although these tend to focus on younger children (Adamson-Macedo, Patel and Sallah 2009; Seeff-Gabriel, Chiat and Roy 2008; Gardner *et al.* 2006; see also the indicators list in Appendix 1).

Another approach is to ask people to look for behaviours which might be indicative of a communication difficulty. There are various 'indicators' of communication difficulty which can help non-specialists decide whether a referral for a fuller assessment is necessary (Afasic checklists 1991; Ripley and Barrett 2008). These are most useful when the person using them knows the young person well and has had some training about communication problems. A couple of very simple 'indicators' might be useful.

Ask the child or young person to repeat back in their own words what you have said. This will give insight into what they have understood and can remember. It will also give you an idea of how they can use language.

When adults use complex language:

- Do the children or young people do what is asked of them?
- How do they behave?
- How well do they listen?
- If the language is simplified, does anything change?

Professionals other than speech and language therapists (SLTs) seem to vary in terms of the training they have received about language development (often they have had none) and therefore have limited confidence in identifying communication problems (Letts and Hall 2003), so collaborative work and training is often the best way to increase appropriate identification of children with communication difficulties. We don't yet have any gold standard screening tools.

Standardised assessment

Researchers and clinicians often identify communication problems by using standardised tests which attempt to compare a child's performance with their peers. The materials and tasks are used in a specific and consistent way, so they are often also called 'formal assessments'. Standardised tests aim to provide quantifiable, objective and repeatable measures of language skills. Indeed, in various states in the US, speech language pathologists are required to use at least two standardised tests to identify a communication problem because of the tests' perceived objectivity, but such tests are not without drawbacks. In the UK, the results of standardised tests are often important in determining access to services (Roulstone *et al.* 2008) but if used alone may provide an incomplete or inaccurate picture.

Standardised, norm-referenced tests are designed and developed in a detailed and lengthy process in an attempt to make them as valid and reliable as possible. This means they should assess what they aim to in a consistent way. To achieve this, certain criteria must be met (Friberg 2010, based on McCauley and Swisher 1984):

- The purpose of the assessment should be identified: Will this identify just the presence or absence of a communication problem and/or its nature?

- The tester's qualifications should be explicitly stated; this is important for the validity of the results, which are at risk if the tester is not qualified to adequately interpret them.

- The testing procedures should be sufficiently explained. This is important so the standardisation conditions can be replicated; if they are not, the scores can't accurately be compared to the standardisation sample.

- There must be adequate standardisation (more than 100 in each subgroup), otherwise accurate comparisons can't be made.

- The standardisation sample must be clearly defined, for example in terms of geography, SES (or parent educational level as a proxy), gender, age, ethnicity and whether any of them had communication problems or not. This is important so that the child being assessed can be compared with similar children.

- There must be evidence of item analysis, to make sure assessors test what they are aiming to and are at the right level. A useful standardised test should be both sensitive and specific. Its sensitivity is the accuracy with which it identifies language impairment, and its specificity is the degree to which it identifies normally developing language. (Merrell and Plante 1997)

- Measures such as mean and standard deviation of scores should be included so comparisons can be made between the child being assessed and the standardisation group.

- There should be concurrent validity, so it should get the same results as similar tests.

- There should be predictive validity, so the results predict a difficulty in a real situation.

- Test/retest reliability is important: a child's results should stay stable over time if their skills do.

- Face validity is important: Does it measure what it says it does?

- Inter-rater reliability is also important so the person conducting the assessment should not impact on the results.

Few current assessments of communication skills meet all these criteria – predictive validity was often missing (Friberg 2010) – so it is important to be aware of the strengths and limitations of any that are used. Burgess and Bransby (1990) used all the formal assessments that they were employing to identify communication problems in children with SEBD on a population of typical children. The validity of these tests was confirmed, as the typically developing children scored well above expected levels.

Formal assessments are further criticised that they are biased against children from minority backgrounds because they rely on experiential history as well as vocabulary knowledge (Campbell *et al.* 1997).

Extension testing can add to the validity of a score because it is a way of checking whether a young person 'really' has difficulties in a certain area, which have been identified by the assessment. This is often useful before learning objectives are set.

In order to maintain validity, standardised tests must be used precisely as their authors suggest. The use of individual subtests rather than the whole assessment can invalidate the results and is therefore not accurate enough for diagnostic decisions. However, in practice, few children with SEBD can cope with a whole standardised assessment at once. The main value of standardised assessments is the comparison they allow with other young people of the same age.

Statistical definitions

Standardised scores, which compare a young person's performance to those of a sample of their peers, are more useful than age-equivalent scores (Wiig 1995). Just because an eight-year-old gains an age equivalent of five years on a test, this does not mean that his or her performance is outside the normal range; only a standard score can give that information. Age equivalents also give limited information because development proceeds at different rates, so getting an age equivalent of two at four is much more significant than getting an age equivalent score of eight at ten, although it does also depend on the skills being measured.

Standardised assessments vary in how they define language impairment or communication problems. The lower end of what is considered to be 'typical' varies from one to one-point-five standard deviations below the mean (Spaulding *et al.* 2006). Cohen and Lipsett (1991), in their study of children with unsuspected communication problems, defined language problems as occurring when a child gained scores which were one standard deviation below the mean on two out of seven standardised tests. Others, such as Giddan *et al.* (1996), combined standard scores with 'clinical judgement' to determine whether a communication problem was present. For the diagnosis of SLI, communication skills need to be two standard deviations below the mean. However, these definitions seem to be more traditional than anything else, and where there is an arbitrary cut-off score typically developing children are also likely to be identified as having communication problems. Another issue is whether norms are up-to-date; in some areas many more children score at minus one-point-five than would be expected in a normal distribution (Vance 2009). It is not clear whether this is to do with SES, deterioration in communication skills or other factors.

There are also problems in comparing across tests, as they probably have different normative samples. This means that comparisons of different areas of form, content and use must only be made with caution, as must considerations of verbal versus non-verbal functioning. Similarly, total scores can be misleading if there is a wide variation in individual subtest scores. Often, the way young people complete the task is as interesting as their score. It is also important to take into account the other skills which are necessary in a formal language assessment: attention, motivation, visual and auditory skills and memory may all be necessary, and if they are lacking, the results will be affected.

Standardised assessments are for identifying the presence or absence of a communication difficulty and are therefore not often sensitive enough to identify changes or progress (Huang, Hopkins and Nippold 1997). A child would have to learn at a faster rate than usual to show an improvement in standard scores, and for some children, maintaining the same standard score could be impressive because it means they are not continuing to fall behind their peers.

An artificial situation

Another, often more significant, problem with formal assessment is its artificiality. Formal testing is by its very nature an unusual situation which does not necessarily call for functional language. This is especially true where an assessor has to give instructions in a precise way, and is not allowed to give the young person any feedback, only general encouragement. The assessment situation itself can be unfamiliar and intimidating, and this could also skew the results. Fulk, Brugham and Lohman (1998) reported that children with SEBD experienced more test anxiety than other groups of students, and that their co-operation might be more difficult to gain. Some authors have minimised the amount of formal assessment used in order to reduce children's anxieties. Blager (1979) felt that children who had been abused or neglected were often fearful or resistant to testing, so she only used those tests which required a non-verbal response. It is also assumed that the child is giving of their best and the influence of anxiety may make this unlikely.

Children or young people often find standardised assessments overlong, and they are forced into a passive role. Children are not given opportunities to initiate interactions or have realistic conversations. As the language used in these assessments is artificial, so is that elicited and it may not be representative of how the child might communicate in real situations. Therefore the results may be of limited use in planning programmes of work. To increase ecological validity (the degree to which the results reflect 'real' situations) some standardised tests, especially those for young children, have a parental report measure as well. This brings us back to the importance of triangulation.

As regards children's understanding of language, sometimes their difficulties can only be uncovered through standardised assessment because they often rely on clues from the environment (what others are doing and an adult's unconscious support though extra gesture and simplification, and, of course, routine) and these are absent in a formal testing situation.

Informal assessments

Informal assessments occur in less-formal situations and are not necessarily standardised, but they can still be detailed and systematic. Their major advantage is their flexibility. The most obvious disadvantage of informal assessments is that it is not necessarily possible to compare results to 'norms'. Furthermore, the results of informal assessments may be subjective and therefore unreliable, in the formal sense, in that people may not always give the same response even if the situation is the same. They may also be ineffective in measuring change because of these sorts of variations. If different teachers or foster carers are asked to give a view of the child's communication, there will inevitably be variations in their responses. However, such assessments may be very useful with low functioning individuals, or where it is difficult to gain co-operation. There are also situations where it is not possible to use standardised assessment because modifications have to be made, perhaps because the young person needs to use some form of communication aid.

It is generally recommended that, as well as formal standardised assessment, additional information be gathered to determine whether a child really has a communication problem or not. This is vital with children and young people who have SEBD. Some authors argue that the most useful information about children with SEBD will be found in dynamic-interactive assessment, functional assessment and observational methods (Rock *et al.* 1997). This section will consider the merits of these and other kinds of informal assessments.

Observation

Direct observation of the way a young person uses language in 'real' situations is often one of the most informative types of assessment. Standardised tests can say something about a child's linguistic strengths and weaknesses, but only observations can tell us how the child or young person copes with the communicative demands of their environment. There are various structured observational tools available, or one can carry out an unstructured observation. One major advantage of observation is that it might highlight strengths or weaknesses that hadn't been noticed before. This is particularly the case if the observation is unstructured, although structured observations help to guide and focus an observation onto relevant features. It is necessary to decide whether the observer takes part in the situation, or whether they try to stay inconspicuous. The observer may also alter the situation to see what happens, or just focus on what occurs naturally.

Observation seems deceptively simple, but in practice observation can be very time-consuming and difficult to interpret. It is hard to know whether what you have seen is representative, significant or to what extent the presence of an observer has affected the outcome. However, an awareness of these factors and the development of an alliance between the observer, observed and those who know the young person well, can minimise them. There is also the issue of recording the observations to consider. In order not to forget anything important, recording has to be done at the time or soon after. Videotaping is especially useful, as it allows for assessment of non-verbal as well as verbal cues and it is objective, but it can also be more intrusive than, for example, a small audio recorder. The issue of consent is very relevant here, as often young people are not keen to be videoed or audio-recorded, and this has to be respected.

The Children's Communicative Checklist (Bishop 1998) designed to assess aspects of the use of language, amongst others, is a useful tool because it requires someone with knowledge of the young person, gained through observation over at least three months. The results can then be compared with a standardisation sample.

An observation of a child's interactions with caregivers provides valuable information: it allows communicative styles to be identified, some of which may be more effective than others as regards enabling language and communication development. Important areas to consider are whether there is responsiveness and positivity to the child, and how the adult helps them learn emotional and communication skills. Clearly, this kind of observation can be very stressful for the adults involved, and therefore it should be sensitively handled. Interpreting what is seen is not straightforward, either, and there is no guarantee that what is observed is really representative of ongoing interactions. Carer–child interactions should also be considered in the wider context, as cultural differences will impact on what is observed as well as its interpretation.

Observations in a variety of settings is important. For young children, an observation of play is useful, such as the Social Play Record (White 2006). Observing play not only provides information on verbal and non-verbal communication and interaction, but it also gives clues to other areas of a child's development such as cognitive and emotional development. For example, symbolic pretend play can give indications about how a child's theory of mind is developing. Teddy won't get fed unless the child understands that others may also feel hunger. An empty spoon will only be used to feed teddy if a child has enough symbolic appreciation to realise that an empty spoon can represent a real one with food on it. As language (another symbolic activity) develops, children are gradually able to 'set the scene' in play, with words rather than real props. Language is also used to develop themes or scripts for play (for example going to the doctor, or army games), and to negotiate roles within these themes.

Observing older children in school, in lessons and at play can be very informative, as there is a great deal to be learnt about how to act and communicate in these situations. The Social Communication Profile (Bedford 2008) can be useful for this. Observations in school will provide information about how well the student copes with the demands of the curriculum and if, and how, their communication problems impair learning. It might also provide clues as to strategies that do and don't work for them. However, trying to observe a young person in school can affect everyone else in the room. Other students may be curious and adults can feel threatened; therefore it is important to explain one's aims and expectations of this kind of exercise, and to feed back findings promptly.

One of the disadvantages of observational assessment is that young people need not do what they find difficult. It is often necessary to 'stress' their language skills in order to identify areas of weakness (Lahey 1990). When they are observed in a naturalistic setting, a young person may seem to be able to converse with their peers adequately. However, it may not be until the same young person is observed in class, where the style and vocabulary of the interaction are very different, that it becomes clear that they have communication problems. Another example of this is children with comprehension problems who talk all the time because then they don't have to try and understand what someone else is saying. It would be difficult to identify their communication problems by just observing such an individual.

Getting a language sample

Sometimes children and young people don't say much when they are observed in naturalistic settings, and it is not always clear why this is. If a communication skill isn't seen, this might be because it is difficult or because there was no opportunity to use this skill in the situation observed. Therefore it might also be useful to elicit a language sample which can then be analysed (Crystal, Garman and Fletcher 1976). There are databases to compare samples with, such as the SALT database (see www.saltsoftware. com), but not for UK-English speaking children.

In order to encourage a child or young person to speak, it is important for the adult to avoid a barrage of questions. Being at the same level with younger children and joining in with their play, following their lead can be helpful. Adults should maintain positive, friendly, non-verbal and verbal communication; in other words, smile and get eye contact while not being dismissive of anything the child says. It is best to observe, wait, listen and then respond to their initiatives, or use a minimum of open questions such as 'What did you think of that?' It is more useful to comment rather than question, and obviously important that the adult takes short turns to leave space for the child or young person. 'I like that elephant' is more likely to elicit language than 'What's that called?'

Interestingly, adolescents with and without communication problems say more when asked to explain something (Nippold *et al.* 2008), for example how to use a social networking site. Observations in real settings and elicited samples can be useful to assess the progress a child or young person is making.

Interviews/questionnaires

Interviews are a useful way to gain information, from the young people themselves as well as from others who know them well. However, young people with communication problems may find this kind of investigation particularly difficult because it involves skills they are not proficient in. Nonetheless, interviews may be less daunting than a formal assessment, especially when they are seen as a way of finding out about what the child and young person can do and their views on their communication skills and needs.

The way questions are phrased directly affects the answers received. Descriptive information is far more informative than judgements, so questions should be carefully worded. Open questions such as 'Tell me about a typical day in your life' will get a very different answer than 'Do you have problems talking to people?' Obviously the young person's expressive language skills will also affect the answer. If they have communication problems, they may be able to respond to a question which requires a yes or no answer but not able to formulate a response to an open question.

Interviews may have set questions planned in advance, or they may follow the informant's train of thought. In an unstructured interview, where specific questions are not determined in advance, it is possible to seek examples, descriptions and explanations. In a more structured interview, answering a series of questions can interrupt the respondent's train of thought and make them feel less able to elaborate. A semi-structured interview format is probably most useful, as it has enough structure to ensure that no important questions are forgotten, but also flexibility which allows for responsiveness to the interviewee and for negotiation of meaning to take place, so that both parties can be sure that they understand each other. It is enlightening in itself to use an interview that allows the respondent to answer in his or her own terms.

The process of being interviewed can be therapeutic because someone is willing to listen and try to understand any difficulties faced. This can also be a disadvantage because of the time necessary to do it thoroughly. Much depends on the characteristics of the interviewer, and whether they are able to make the interviewee comfortable enough to be forthcoming and keep them on track. Interviews can, of course, also be intimidating if not carried out sensitively. Another important issue with questionnaires or interviews is their subjectivity, so in the triangulation of views between home and school, for example, there are often different views on whether behaviour is acceptable or whether social communication skills are adequate or not. No doubt this depends on the adults being interviewed, but it also depends on the context in which they see the children and young people. Obviously parents do have a longitudinal perspective unavailable to professionals, but of course they don't necessarily see children and young people in comparison to large groups of peers. The Pragmatics Profile (Dewart and Summers 1995) can be useful for interviewing parents, carers and teachers to gather information about a child's social communication skills.

Criterion referenced assessment

Criterion referenced assessments can be used to see how a pupil performs in response to specific situational demands. An example of this is whether they know and can use the vocabulary required for a history project, in particular, words ending in '–ism' (colonialism, racism, etc.). It is also possible to assess how much of a lesson a pupil understood and retained by observing the lesson then talking to them about it afterwards. These types of assessments can be used to identify features of communication difficulties which are not assessed by formal assessments (Bishop 1998). Criterion referenced tests are useful once communication problems have been identified but would not necessarily help to identify communication problems. These are also useful where norm referenced tests are not available, where the standardisation is not appropriate or where information about very specific language skills is needed (McCauley 1996).

There are various curriculum-based criterion-referenced assessments in England (National Curriculum Key Stage One and Two attainment targets in English (Department for Education and Skills 2003), and Assessing Pupils' Progress (APP) in English) that can be used to monitor pupils' progress. However, by its very nature, criterion reference assessments like these do not indicate when a pupil has a communication problem or is developing typically.

Dynamic assessment

Dynamic assessment is an assessment of the ability to learn language rather than of language learnt. It is useful because it gives some indication of the young person's potential. Dynamic assessment considers what a young person can do, with and without support, and how they learn. Sometimes young people have communication problems because they have not had opportunities to learn the relevant skills rather than because they are unable to learn these skills, and dynamic assessment can help to differentiate these two groups of young people. Such assessment might be particularly useful to identify those with communication problems when a child is learning more than one language (Camilleri and Law 2007). The nature of bilingualism varies in terms of how, when and by whom languages are used in the child's context, so not only is it often difficult to access suitably trained translators but also very difficult to decide whether a child's progress is indicative of a communication difficulty.

It is possible to use dynamic assessment to assess a child's narrative abilities and thereby identify those with communication problems (Peña *et al.* 2006). This involves teaching a narrative skill that the child has not yet acquired – perhaps the importance of including the setting, or the character's response to events – and then observing how well the child is able to learn and use these skills. Children who do not have communication problems can easily improve their narratives with such individual support, but those who do often need much more focused, individual help. Dynamic assessment has also been shown to be useful in highlighting information useful for intervention (Hasson and Botting 2010).

Assessing the communicative environment

The child or young person may have communication problems, but they will succeed or fail in an interaction depending on their conversational partner and what's expected of them. It is therefore important to also consider how responsive the conversational partner is, and how well they adapt their speech to the young person in order to help them succeed. We also need to think carefully about the tasks presented to young people, in school and in order to help them learn emotional and behavioural skills. Are these modified so the language is accessible to young people? Some ways of evaluating the communicative environment are available (Ealing Quality Indicators 2010; and as part of I CAN's talk programmes – see www.ican.org.uk/en/what-we-do.aspx).

Conclusion

There are various informal and formal methods of assessing language skills, all of which have advantages and disadvantages. No individual method is likely to provide a satisfactory assessment of a child's communication skills and indeed relying on standardised formal assessment could be misleading. The most useful assessment of communication skills is likely to be one which uses a variety of strategies, including formal and informal methods, and which assesses form, content and use in various situations. This should be able to identify a communication problem and its nature in order to inform intervention. We are a long way from being able to offer a firm prognosis; a great deal of further research is necessary before we can even identify who is at most risk, although those with SEBD are likely to benefit from even the recognition of their communication problems.

Chapter 6

What Can be Done to Help Young People with Communication, Emotional and Behavioural Problems?

Introduction

Despite the considerable adversities some children with SEBCD have experienced and the limited skills they may have, it is still possible for them to learn and develop positively. The more we learn about the plasticity of the brain and its potential (Doidge 2008), particularly in the right environment, the more hope there is. Although more research into interventions is necessary, we know enough to successfully help many of these children and young people. Children with SEBCD have serious implications for service delivery, and helping them develop language skills should probably be considered as a public health issue (Law and Elliott 2009).

However, 'For every complex problem there is an answer that is clear, simple, and wrong' (Mencken 1917). Young people with SEBCD are often challenging and lead to a clamour for 'strategies' to apply from the adults around them. However, the application of many clever ideas has failed because the first and most important step – really understanding why this behaviour occurs – has been omitted. Strategies are more likely to work if they are used as the result of a careful assessment or knowing the child well. For a successful answer to a complex problem, professionals, the young people and their family or carers need to share their insights with each other, and work together to form and carry out a plan of action.

Another issue which impedes progress for children with SEBCD is the lack of 'experts'. However, it is not necessary to be trained as an SLT, psychologist or psychotherapist to make communication and behaviour easier for these children and young people, although of course their contributions are very valuable. The first section in this chapter discusses things that anyone can do, changes we can make as adults and communication and interaction skills we can all teach and encourage in children and young people.

The second section includes information on specific interventions which have potential for children with SEBCD. It must be stressed that what follows is by no means an exhaustive list of possible interventions; neither can any specific intervention be described in detail here. Rather, it is simply an overview of the types of intervention which have proved useful in working with young people with SEBCD.

Since communication problems and SEBD often develop together, there is the possibility of interventions which could address both difficulties. Laplante *et al.* (1991) trained parents to manage their children's oppositional behaviour and found that as the misbehaviour decreased, vocabulary and verbal interaction increased in comparison with controls. 'The more we create the right kind of environment for our children with good relationships and appropriate stimulation, the more angels we create and the fewer rogues' (Perry 2004, cited in Sinclair 2007, p.18).

What everyone can do to support children and young people with SEBCD
The role of the adult
POSITIVE RESPONSIVE INTERACTIONS

The interaction style that children need in order to develop their social, emotional, behavioural and communication skills mirrors that in a secure attachment. It is accepting, genuine and empathic (Rogers 1961). Therefore the relationship in itself can be as useful as any specific interventions for young people with SEBCD. Some adults are anxious about forming attachments with the children they work with; they imagine the child as a limpet they won't be able to shake off, and others worry about adults becoming over involved with children. We cannot replace original attachment figures, but we can show children and young people that positive and supportive relationships are possible. What is important is knowing the children well, and understanding their patterns of attachment in order to make our intervention more effective. Warm relationships where school staff show respectful and empathic compassionate concern are part of what makes a school effective in supporting children's mental health (Nind and Weare 2009).

The components of positive interactions have been characterised in various ways; one is the PRIDE model (Gershenson, Lyon and Budd 2010). Ways in which this might be relevant to children with SEBCD are presented in Table 6.1.

Table 6.1 PRIDE model		
Skill	Why?	Examples
PRAISE appropriate behaviour.	This helps develop a positive interaction and is likely to encourage the behaviour being praised.	'I loved the way you let him join in the conversation.'
REFLECT appropriate speech.	This shows that you have listened and heard and provides opportunities to model more complex language.	Child: 'I made a castle.' Adult: 'Yes, you made a gloomy castle.'
IMITATE appropriate behaviour/play.	The child gets attention for positive behaviour and this can increase co-operation.	Child is drawing. Adult begins to doodle.
DESCRIBE appropriate behaviour.	The child knows what they are doing well and that this behaviour gets positive adult attention.	'You are listening to him and taking turns!'
Be ENTHUSIASTIC in tone and body language.	This adds to the positivity of the interaction and increases interest in the participants.	Adult uses a playful tone and inflection with frequent smiles.

The PRIDE model needs to be modified for older children, but many of the key elements are still useful. When an adult follows a child's lead, this gets the child's attention. They realise they have an adult's attention, and that they are interested. The effects of this are that children are often more willing to interact and co-operate with the adult. They may begin to realise that trying to communicate is worth it because their attempts will be 'received'. They have learnt that interactions can be positive. Adults show interest and respect by actively listening to a child or young person's point of view and concerns. In an effective, enjoyable interaction, both partners take short turns and no one dominates the conversation. In practice this often requires the adult to say less and offer more opportunities for the child or young person to have a turn. There may be conscious and unconscious mirroring of behaviours which is evidence of attunement.

Through understanding children's intentions it is possible for the adult to help them learn. The best way to support learning is to provide just enough support in a new task for them to succeed, then to gradually withdraw it as they develop their skills. This is known as 'scaffolding' (Vygotsky 1962). In order to provide good scaffolding, adults need to be alert and responsive to the children's level of skill and need for support and to have gained their trust.

Providing 'language stimulation' will be less effective if it is not in the context of a responsive interaction (van Balkom *et al.* 2010). Sensitive and stimulating interactions with teachers lead to the most gains in language and other skills (Burchinalab *et al.* 2008). To take it to its extreme, it is possible to learn the 'language' of those without verbal communication, through responsive and interactive intensive interaction, and thereby increase joint attention and reduce behavioural difficulties (Zeedyk 2008).

Positive interactions are enjoyable; many children with SEBCD have had few good experiences, so even a brief conversation that makes them feel good is very valuable. Where interactions between carers and children become more positive, children's language skills also improve (Evangelou *et al.* 2005). It may be difficult to be positive about someone whose behaviour is challenging, but trying to understand what they have experienced and the difficulties they currently face might help to reframe their actions. As adults we have to remember how those who behave well and have sunny dispositions get more positive interactions and therefore more opportunities to learn language, emotional and social interaction skills. The adult can turn the tide of negativity to which many children and young people with SEBD are exposed by finding the positives in them. A clear distinction needs to be made between responses to the young person and to the way they behave. It is possible to be non-judgemental of young people but not necessarily of their behaviour. An important part of this positivity is believing that the child or young person can make progress, expressing this, and pointing out small steps forward. A sense of belief in the young person can become a self-fulfilling prophecy. Moods are catching, and the adult often has more resources to lighten the mood or see the positives in a difficult situation. When this happens, it is often greatly appreciated by young people (Johnson 2008). It is also possible to increase approving comments after a short training, and this has a positive impact on children's behaviour (Swinson and Harrop 2005).

Trust is a key component of a positive interaction. Setting clear limits to behaviour is part of this; it can take time, and boundaries will be tested, but ultimately clear limits on behaviour lead to a sense of security. Part of this, for children with SEBCD is knowing that an adult is honest and consistent. The limits of the relationship may have to be defined. An adult may have to explain to a young person that they'd feel more comfortable if the young person said, 'Hello, how are you?' rather than using hugging as a greeting in school. They may have to explain that 'It's my job to help you in school, not outside of it'. Making these sort of expectations explicit will also help a child or young person with social communication skills to interact more appropriately. Confidentiality within the adult–young person interaction also helps to build trust. The young person needs to know what confidentiality means, how far it extends and when it might be broken (usually only if a child protection issue arises). If confidentiality has to be broken, then the young person has to be informed and told why.

Butler and Williamson (1994) found that young people in the care of the local authority want professionals to listen, be available, be non-judgemental and non-directive. They also valued adults with a sense of humour, who were honest and trustworthy. While humour is very important, sarcasm can be very detrimental to a positive relationship, not least because young people with communication difficulties may take it literally and be puzzled and offended. Those who can use humour tend to be more resilient (Werner and Smith 1992), so it's a good skill to foster.

As regards older children and young people, positive interactions could be summarised thus:

- Listen.
- Believe them.
- Take a genuine interest.
- Give honest feedback.
- Take outside pressures into account.
- Respect what they say.
- Use their name more often.
- End on a positive.

BEING AN EMOTIONAL COACH

If the ability to read emotions is built on the empathy we are shown as children, the same is true as children grow into young people. Adults have to continue to be emotional coaches. This is, of course, not just learning about emotions but also the language to describe and discuss them.

Zeidner, Matthews and Roberts (2009, p.158) suggest that emotional coaching needs to include the following:

- Explain complex emotions.

- Direct to key emotional cues.

- Point out consequences.

- Help the child understand and manage their responses.

- Segment social interactions to explain emotions.

When a child is upset:

- Redirect thoughts and attention.

- Use positive self-talk.

- Redefine goals or outcomes.

Emotional coaching is essentially really trying to understand how a child or young person feels without imposing your own ideas, eventually helping them find the words to describe and understand it. It is helpful to try to name emotions as they occur, in a tentative way, for example 'I wonder if that made you jealous' or 'You look like you might be getting angry... Are you?' There may well be core feelings which are not so obvious, so what appears to be anger could really be sadness. When you know someone well, you may get some insight into these things. It is vital that no one is ever compelled to talk about their feelings but that they are offered opportunities to do so and chances to hear about other people's feelings. Encourage the children or young people to think about other people's feelings and how they affect the way they behave; stories, TV and films provide good opportunities for this.

Calm interventions are best in any emotional situation, alongside an acknowledgement of the feelings being expressed either verbally or non-verbally. Feelings need to be validated. Obviously it is acceptable to experience all emotions, but only some ways of expressing them are acceptable (and this will vary from society to society). We would often prefer that children and young people said how they felt rather than acted it out through inappropriate behaviour. Modelling clear expression of emotions such as 'I feel sad when you talk to him like that' is therefore useful.

Having discussions about how we can 'manage' our emotions is also vital for a child or young person's emotional development. Examples of this are ways we can cheer ourselves up, get over disappointment and, most importantly, calm ourselves. It can come as a great relief for a young person to realise that we all struggle with difficult feelings at times, and we have various ways of managing them. Again it is important not to impose ideas but to suggest them; we all do this differently. Part of this is discussing what we say to ourselves in difficult situations. Children and young people may think, 'It's hopeless, I'm useless, I never get anything right, I should give up'. But adults can explain they could also try thinking, ' I made a mistake'; 'Just because it's bad now doesn't mean it'll be bad forever'; 'I can do it'; 'I can try'; 'Sometimes other people and the situation make it harder for me.' This is known as positive self-talk and it can have a huge impact. It is part of what is addressed in cognitive behaviour therapy (CBT).

Moments of upset can be used as opportunities to talk about what it feels like and what options there are for making it feel better, accepting it or reframing it. These moments are also important because, by talking about them, adults can show that emotions needn't be overwhelming; they can be 'contained'. These discussions should always happen after someone has had time to calm down. When very distressed, the 'thinking' brain is not really working and too much talk from others can increase the stress.

Adults working with young people who have SEBCD also have to consider their own emotional awareness. They must be able to tolerate the strong and distressing emotions that the young person may express. In response to these negative emotions, adults should avoid retaliation and show an ability to bear frustrations – and realise that it's unreasonable to expect gratitude for having done this. Any negative behaviour directed at an adult may not really be about that adult, though sometimes it can be difficult not to take it personally.

Emotions are contagious. Our mood can affect the children and young people we work with, and their feelings will affect us. As adults we may also experience strong responses to a young person because of our own past experiences. We need to recognise when something in our past interferes with our interactions with young people. We might respond to children behaving inappropriately in one way because they remind us of someone we loved, and in another if they are like someone we hated. It is important to try and understand this, particularly in a relationship with a 'difficult' child. The young people's feelings can be transferred to an adult working with them or another young person. This can make the adult feel as hurt and confused as the young people do, unless they understand what this transference of emotion is. The adults in a situation like this need to be able to survive this onslaught then try to help the young person understand what is going on. Adults can help young people with SEBCD by being aware of where the strong feelings are coming from and by encouraging the appropriate expression of such emotions.

This links to an important psychotherapeutic idea: 'using one's own feelings as a barometer, not only of how one is feeling, but also what is going on for others; what you are picking up from others' (Whitwell 2002). Adults can develop their ability to be 'mindful': aware of a wider perspective of what is happening in the present for oneself and others through meditation. This increased awareness of psychological, physical and emotional sensations can lead to a growth in the brain (Lazar *et al.* 2005) and increase resistance to disease (Lutz, Dunne and Davidson 2007). It may also be a useful intervention for children and young people (Black, Milam and Sussman 2009).

There is another section in this chapter (p.136) on teaching emotional literacy skills, but being an emotional coach is something that can happen outside of specific lessons and activities. It can happen any time and anywhere, and because it allows for discussion about emotions as they happen, it has enormous potential for helping children and young people develop their emotional skills and communication skills. It also provides opportunities for adults to praise and reinforce a child or young person when they begin to use these skills.

MODIFYING YOUR LANGUAGE

The communicative style of the person a child or young person interacts with will influence the development of their communication skills (Duchan 1989). In order to facilitate language development, it is useful to avoid a directive style but rather to follow their lead and talk about that. Language development occurs in 'real' conversations where the adult does not try to control its direction but builds on the child's contributions. Responding to a child or young person's attempts to initiate conversation is key, even if it is only to say 'I can't talk to you right now'.

Given that children and young people with communication problems may have difficulty processing and understanding what they hear, adults talking with them have a responsibility to express themselves in an accessible way. As many as 37 per cent of teacher instructions in some schools contain multiple meanings, 20 per cent with at least one idiom, such as 'shake a leg' (Lazar et al. 1989). Avoiding or explaining complex vocabulary enables comprehension. Simple, direct statements are easiest to understand, though they are often rare in adult speech.

It may also be necessary to slow one's rate of speech and to reduce the length and complexity of sentences. Pausing between phrases will allow time for processing. These things are much easier said than done, and it is useful to have feedback to develop these skills, either from the listeners or through using video or audio recording.

As auditory input may be problematic for a young person with communication difficulties, giving additional visual or kinaesthetic support can be very helpful. Pictures, diagrams and practical activities, alongside spoken explanations, will often be far more effective than talking alone. See the Symbols Inclusion Project website for ideas – www. symbolsinclusionproject.org.

In order to overcome comprehension or vocabulary learning difficulties, it is important to repeat key information and concepts often. If someone has attention difficulties, saying his or her name to get attention before starting to say anything will reduce the number of failed attempts at communication. You can stress the importance of listening by refusing to talk until you are being listened to, but that can take a long time. Adults also have a very important role to play in encouraging young people to say when they don't understand. There are times when we all have difficulty following what someone says, and one can be a good role model by saying so and asking for clarification.

If a child or young person is having difficulty expressing themselves, an adult's focused attention is invaluable. Some children and young people may not be able to use spoken language and will rely on signing or symbols, in which case adults will need a familiarity with the system they are using in addition to the following strategies. Young people with expressive difficulties may simply need more time to formulate and express an idea, so patience is vital. In this situation, adults may a have a greater role in keeping the conversation going, the most effective way being to comment and pause to allow for a response rather than bombarding the children with questions. Respond to what they say, or the emotions being expressed, not how they say it. It is important not to 'correct' but to provide models of how to say it in your response, so if a child says, 'he goed', an adult could say, 'Oh, he went, did he?' However, if it were the first time the child had ever put two words together, it would be more appropriate to accept the communication unconditionally (and with much excitement).

Another useful strategy is called 'expanding'; if a child produces a short or incomplete sentence, the adult can respond using the same sentences but expanding it slightly. For example, if the young person says, 'He went out, he went to school', the adult could suggest, 'He went out because it was time for school?' It is also possible to model the required language; for example, if someone is getting angry about not being heard, an adult could suggest the child say, 'Excuse me, can I tell you about it from my point of view?' etc. Keeping on topic may also be difficult, and adults can help redirect those who wander. Similarly, if a young person gives too much or too little information this can be pointed out by saying things like 'Yes, I saw that', or 'Who are you talking about?' A good relationship between young people and the adult will enable the adult to know which strategies are likely to be acceptable and when to offer them.

The type of questions used can also influence how much a young person joins in a conversation. Open questions such as 'What do you think about that?' are likely to encourage more of a response than 'Did you like that?' However, if the child has difficulty formulating sentences or narratives, it might be easier for them not to try to answer open questions. Then it can be useful to offer alternatives: 'Was it funny or was it boring?' Obviously you are also narrowing possible responses when you do this, so it's important to be aware of this. As adults we sometimes ask very odd questions such as, 'What is that?' when we know what it is and the child knows that we know, too. Such questions are not as helpful as those which are genuine.

Listening to and telling stories is key to our experience as humans. Almost every conversation we have includes anecdotes or recounts of events. We enjoy this, and it helps us connect with each other. Making opportunities to include children and young people in storytelling is useful in many ways. We know that those who have difficult beginnings are able to move on from them if they can construct a narrative about it. Therefore listening to and telling stories, recounting shared events, reading together and talking about the emotions, problems and consequences in a story all help develop language and emotional skills.

Appendix 2 has more detail of strategies to support children and young people with various communication problems.

ENABLING APPROPRIATE BEHAVIOUR

There are many schools of thought which contribute ideas about how to improve children's behaviour, briefly summarised below:

- Systemic: considers the child in the context of the family, the school, the wider system of people who support them and how they all interact. See Dallos and Draper (2010).

- Behavioural: assumes behaviour is learnt through reinforcement, so it modifies behaviour through rewards, sanctions and the identification of triggers.

- Cognitive: recognises how thoughts influence feelings and actions. Reframes negative and unhelpful thoughts, focuses on the here and now. See Kennerly (2009) and Royal College of Psychiatrists (2008).

- Therapeutic: attachment theory, how past experiences can continue to affect us, the conscious and unconscious effect of emotions. See Music (2011).

Most practitioners use ideas from all of these schools of thought, and anyone working with children with SEBCD needs to be familiar with them. Anyone using any of these types of interventions should consider how the possibility of the child or young person having communication problems could affect the approach. Clearly, having difficulty understanding or using language (or, indeed, with social communication skills) will affect a young person's access to and the success of any intervention. However, language competence is rarely evaluated before a child undertakes verbally based interventions (Cohen 2003), and we don't know how effective such interventions might be if the child or young person has communication problems.

The language component of any intervention programme for children with SEBD should be modified appropriately for children who also have communication problems. Any rules or expectations must make sense to those who are expected to follow them, there should not be too many of them, they should be positively stated (for example 'Walk away if you're angry' rather than 'Don't hit Jim') and the language must be accessible to those it applies to. The same applies to behaviour policies in general: behaviours and their consequences need to be clear, which might be difficult to achieve if children and young people have difficulty understanding sequences or time vocabulary. This is particularly important when the behaviour is extreme. Recent guidance on the use of force (Department for Children, Schools and Families 2010b, point 37) states, 'Before using force, staff should engage the pupil in a calm and measured tone, making clear that their behaviour is unacceptable and setting out how the pupil could choose to change their behaviour'. Plainly, in a situation like this, it is imperative that the language used is not too complex for the child or young person to understand; but given what we know about undetected communication problems, can we be sure this is always the case?

We must never forget the devastating impact attachment difficulties and living in difficult circumstances can have on a child's emotional and behavioural development, and the many other reasons why inappropriate behaviour arises. However, I want to focus on the role of communication in enabling appropriate behaviour. What is often overlooked is that for those with SEBCD a whole range of strategies to improve communication and interactions can improve behaviour. For example, in severely impaired young people, providing functional communication reduces behavioural problems (Durand and Merges 2001). These strategies are often helpful for all children and young people.

Some key ideas are:

- Prevention is best. Are adult interactions with the child as positive and enabling as they can be? A difficult situation can often be defused by adults really listening to the child's or young person's concerns. In order to prevent behavioural issues it is important to know what skills the child has; there may be gaps in communication and emotional skills that make it difficult for him or her to do what is required. Are adults modifying what they say and ask in relation to any communication skills gaps? Are they teaching the communication and emotional skills children need to behave well?

- Try to understand why this behaviour is occurring. Amongst all the other potential causes of behavioural issues, an often neglected basis is that children and young people might not have the necessary communication skills. They may not be able to understand what is being asked of them, explain their point of view, manage their emotions or interact appropriately. Anyone faced with the impossible will get frustrated and may not behave well as a result. Young people's inappropriate behaviour may make sense to them because they are trying to solve a problem; our job is to help them do that in another way. Inappropriate behaviour is a form of communication, so it is crucial to be able to identify the communicative function of that behaviour, or what the young person is trying to 'say'. Careful observation and often video recording is necessary in order to untangle this.

- Offer opportunities to learn the skills necessary for behaving well. Communication skills are often lacking in those who don't behave in acceptable ways. Once we know this, we can teach children how to express themselves with words rather than unacceptable behaviour. This is often involves teaching things like how to take a turn, phrases to use to ask to join in and ways to express emotions or negotiate.

So we need to ask ourselves:

- Am I being impatient, or expecting too much? Does the child or young person have the communicative and emotional skills to do what I'm asking? Does he or she need extra time to process or plan communication?

- Do they really understand what they are being asked to do?

- Is this young person trying to communicate something but does not know how?

- Have I made clear what I want them to do or say instead of the unacceptable behaviour?

- Have I tried to understand what it is like for them, for example not understanding what is going to happen next?

- Have I supported what I'm saying with visual cues or examples, particularly at times of transition between activities? Do they have access to visual ways to signal 'I don't understand'; or 'I'm getting upset/angry/distracted?'

- If the children or young people are not engaged in what I'd like them to do, is the task inappropriate in terms of language?

Many difficult behaviours can be 'nipped in the bud' by a gentle reminder of what's necessary, tactical ignoring or distraction, or by praising the appropriate behaviour.

In the midst of a crisis, everyone can be upset and it is even harder to process language. So in order to de-escalate:

- Listen carefully and actively.

- Stay calm: don't smile, try to force eye contact or speak loudly; try to keep your body language relaxed and non-confrontational.

- Acknowledge their point of view.

- Apologise for anything that was unjust: 'I'm sorry that's how it felt'.

- Agree with even the smallest bit of truth in what they say.

- Keep your language to a minimum, for example 'You stop shouting, then we can sort it out'.

- Offer a compromise, or choices of ways to solve the problem.

- Don't try to talk things through; do that later.

In trying to deal with difficult behaviour it is important to avoid action without thought, because that is what those behaving inappropriately are doing. Someone wise once said to me, 'They can teach us to be inappropriate quicker than we can teach them to be appropriate'. One needs to bear in mind that the only thing we can control in a difficult situation is ourselves, and our responses are important.

We have to be careful that the way in which we manage inappropriate behaviour is not counterproductive. Time out from a social situation may be just what children with communication problems want; and they then lose out on opportunities to learn how to interact well. Similarly if an intervention results in one-to-one time with an adult, this can be just what a child wants. We need to find ways to give them one-to-one time when they are behaving well, so they don't resort to unacceptable behaviour to get it.

Beware of complex explanations of consequences or sanctions. Where adults focus on behaviour and dominate turn-taking, children use restricted and less complex language (Girolametto, Weitzman and van Lieshart 2000). Some young people will not be able to understand the language and ideas involved in injunctions like 'If you don't do that writing, you will lose your break', or 'Hit him again and you'll go to bed'. It is therefore important to keep language simple and use other ways to explain, such as diagrams or flow charts.

Children and young people with SEBCD may benefit from specific teaching of social problem-solving skills, with simple language and visual support such as solving problems with words (see Figure 6.1). This sort of structure helps them see the other person's point of view, think carefully about what they could do to solve the problems and consider the consequences of potential solutions.

1. Listen.

2. Think about people's feelings.

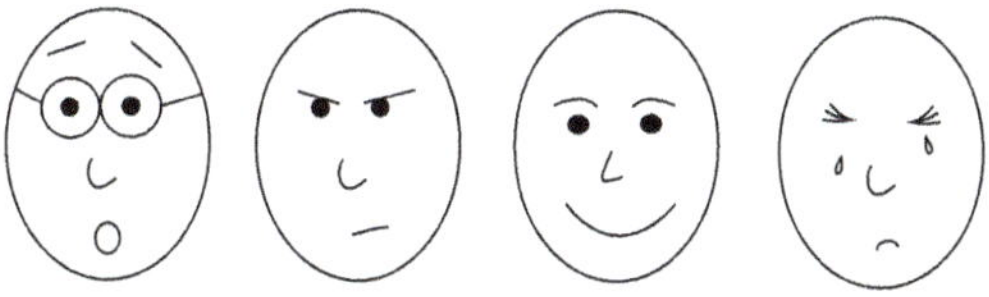

3. How could you solve the problem?

    a.

    b.

    c.

4. What might happen if you try these?

    a.

    b.

    c.

5. What is the best choice?

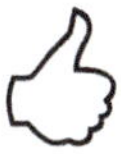

Aim for win-win so everyone is OK.

Figure 6.1 Solving problems with words

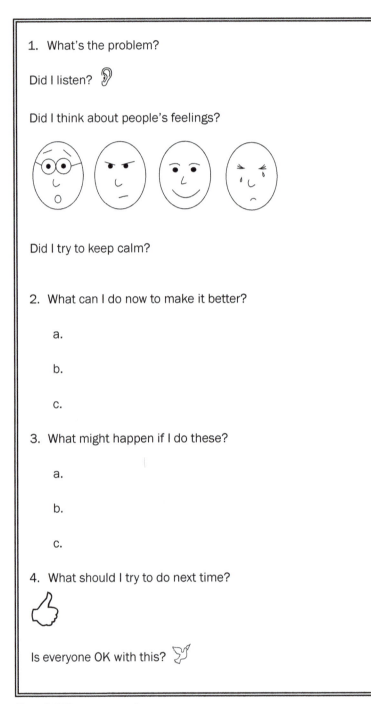

Figure 6.2 What went wrong?

Then if problems occur, when the children are calm they can use a similar form to debrief and think about what happened (see Figure 6.2).

Self-observation and self-monitoring of positive behaviours often serve to improve behaviour generally; these skills also raise self-esteem and lead to a growing sense of responsibility. Children and young people can be given a cue to prompt monitoring, and then they decide if they are achieving their behavioural aim at that point. It may be something like 'Am I listening?' or 'Am I following instructions?' This sort of self-monitoring can increase attention to task (Gureasko-Moore, Dupaul and White 2006). Young people can also monitor and mentor each other, as regards the right kinds of interactions. Video feedforward, where children see video of themselves being successful (through careful editing), is also useful for developing reading (Dowrick, Kim-Rupnow and Power 2006) and social interaction skills.

Social stories (Gray 1994) are designed to provide young people with accurate and specific social information about situations that they find difficult. Each story starts with detailed information about the setting. The person writing the story must try to see the problematic situation from the young person's point of view. The story contains three types of sentences. The descriptive sentences describe the social situation; the perspective sentences describe how other people view the situation, their reactions, responses and feelings; and the directive sentences describe how people ought to respond to this situation or the desired response in this situation. The stories' visual and static nature can help a young person learn relevant cues and common responses. Social stories have been shown to be effective with children with SEBCD (Schneider 2009), helping them stay on task. Comic strip conversations (Gray 1994) work in a similar way, helping young people see other people's perspectives; they can be used to help pupils think through problematic situations, perhaps where their own behaviour deteriorated.

So key strategies for children and young people with SEBCD are:

- Think about what function the behaviour serves.
- Model appropriate language alternatives to challenging behaviours.
- Provide opportunities to teach emotional language.
- Involve peers and parents.

(Nungesser and Watkins 2005)

WORKING IN COLLABORATION

No one profession has all the skills to help children and young people with SEBCD. These children often have complex needs which require support from many adults, including, of course, their parents and carers. For this support to be effective, these adults need to collaborate.

All adults who regularly have conversations with a child or young person can gather information about his or her SEBCD to contribute to an assessment and work together to decide how to approach any communication difficulties found. This is, of course, often easier said than done. Another major barrier to effective teamwork is the considerable shortages of trained professionals in some areas.

Collaboration is not always easy because of the divisive pressures within systems and because people can feel threatened and undermined by the perceived roles and expectations of others. Negotiation of roles and responsibilities is therefore a crucial part of the process of collaboration. It may be useful to formalise the process by using a trans-disciplinary problem analysis framework (Woolfson *et al.* 2003). The first stage of this is to establish roles and expectations, then to think about guiding hypotheses and how information will be gathered. Through this process, a joint problem analysis and action plan can be achieved. This is superior to many professionals doing separate assessments and trying to work separately with the child or young person and their family. In order to increase efficiency and holistic working, a trans-disciplinary model is recommended by the Royal College of Speech and Language Therapists (Gascoigne 2006).

What makes collaboration feasible is having the time in which to do it. There needs to be opportunities to share knowledge and skills (Palikara *et al.* 2007). Evidence about collaboration between teachers and SLTs shows that it is most effective when those involved have a clear understanding of each other's roles, when SLTs take account of the educational context, where teachers understand the importance of language to the whole curriculum and where schools support SLTs' involvement (Law *et al.* 2000). Collaboration can lead to good outcomes for children with SEBCD (Cross *et al.* 2001; Law and Sivyer 2003).

Not all professionals receive formal 'emotional' supervision, as opposed to professional supervision which is often about monitoring competence. So supporting each other is an important part of collaboration. People working with children or young people with SEBD often need emotional support to cope with the challenges they face. Supportive colleagues are useful to help understand and process difficult feelings and to help generate solutions.

KEEP LEARNING

Interdisciplinary training seems to be an important element when it comes to helping children with complex needs. Academia and the professions are divided into 'subject' areas, but children are not. Learning alongside different disciplines not only helps in understanding their theoretical viewpoint but also the practical and organisational difficulties they face. Professionals need to be aware of the terminology and the legal and practical contexts in which others work.

Mental health issues and communication problems need to be highlighted in the training of all professionals working with young people with SEBD, as this is not currently the case. An I CAN YouGov poll of 349 teachers found that only 27 per cent had received training about communication problems, and 81 per cent felt they would benefit from more training on this issue (The Communication Trust 2010). There is a need for much more training around mental health issues, as it can be difficult to determine which behaviours stem from them and which relate to SEN (Rose *et al.* 2009).

It is often difficult for teachers to identify children with communication problems (Antoniazzi, Snow and Dickson-Swift 2010). So an important part of any training would be an awareness of typical development and the identification of communication problems and how to support these young people. Teachers' confidence in working with children with communication problems can be increased though training (Paradice *et al.* 2007). The Speech, Language and Communication Framework (The Communication Trust undated) is a useful online audit of skills and knowledge in speech, language and communication which is designed for anyone working with children and which provides pointers to further training. The Inclusion Development Programme (Department for Children, Schools and Families 2008c) is an online continuing development resource which helps teachers work with pupils who have various special needs, including speech, language and communication needs and SEBD.

SLTs may need more training about SEBD and mental health issues than they currently receive. Some feel that they have insufficient training to work with children with SEBD (Parow 2009). However, in this same study, one significant factor was that school staff did not see communication difficulties as a priority. Ostrov and Godleski (2007) provides SLTs with social development indicators for referrals to mental health professionals, but more joint training with other professionals would be useful. Research suggest that effective continuing professional development occurs when:

- the individual is involved in identifying their learning needs
- it is planned, personalised and evaluated
- it models evidence based, effective learning and teaching strategies
- it is supported by coaching or mentoring
- it uses specialist input
- it involves practical activity in the workplace
- it involves critical reflection.

(Berquez et al. *2009)*

Teach young people skills

Adults can encourage the development of key skills in children and young people with SEBCD by providing scaffolding while they learn and teaching specific skills. What young people can do today with help they can do by themselves tomorrow (Gallagher 1999).

EMOTIONAL LITERACY

As we have seen, there are strong links between the ability to understand emotions and positive behaviour (Ensor and Hughes 2005), so emotional literacy skills are important to teach. A starting point might be to use an emotional literacy assessment; an interesting initial discussion can be about the different perspectives a child, their parent/s and their teachers may have on this (Faupel 2003).

Way *et al.* (2007) provide ideas on how to help children link their physical state with emotions such as through encouraging them to think about their heart rate and learning calming strategies. The use of heart rate monitors has also been helpful in identifying how the emotional states of individuals in families and schools can affect each other and how, if adults want children to change, they may need to change first (McHugh *et al.* 2010). Similarly the use of emotion scales where children rate their feelings can be helpful (see Figure 6.3).

Figure 6.3 How I feel now

They can also use scales to rate emotions which help them learn the appropriate vocabulary, for example: Are you peeved/irritated/annoyed/wound up/angry/furious/fuming/irate/livid/enraged/incensed?

Name: Ben

10	How does it feel to be out of control?
9	no thinking tense hot
8	heart racing shouting
7	
6	
5	Get a grip strategies if my number is going up: 1. Have time out alone 2. Chill out on a bean bag
4	
3	
2	
1	How does it feel to be calm?
0	I can sort things out relaxed happy

Where are you now?

Figure 6.4 Emotion thermometer

Emotion thermometers can be used to help a young person rate how stressed they are by putting an arrow on a 1–10 scale (see Figure 6.4). They can then relate this to calm and very upset feelings. Part of the process of developing an individual emotion thermometer with young people is helping them to think about strategies they can use to calm themselves, their 'get a grip' strategies. Key to this is their recognition of their emotional temperature rising; so when it gets above five, they may need to start using their get a grip strategies.

There are resources available to help children identify emotional cues such as mindreading software (Wheelwright and Baron-Cohen 2007) and *The Transporters* DVD (available from www.thetransporters.com).

Activities like a worry box (where you put all the things you might need to talk about on slips of paper) or an emotion tree (where everyone puts up how they feel) all put emotions on the agenda for discussion and reinforce their significance in everyday life. Teaching simple mindfulness and relaxation skills can also be useful for children and young people. Research shows that being able to calm oneself is a vital emotional tool (Seligman 2006).

The Promoting Alternative Thinking Strategies (PATHS) curriculum, (Greenberg *et al.* 1995) is an emotional literacy curriculum which has had a positive effect on children's development. Interestingly, one of its effects is that it can improve verbal fluency (Riggs *et al.* 2006); the authors therefore recommend that programmes designed to develop social emotional skills should also explicitly develop language skills.

The Social and Emotional Aspects of Learning (SEAL) resources provide a framework for teaching social, emotional and behavioural skills in school. Although it is a great resource, the language is sometimes too complex and needs to be simplified for pupils with communication problems. There is evidence that small group work based on SEAL can have an impact on the development of pupils' social and emotional skills (Humphrey *et al.* 2008). Although a recent review of the secondary SEAL programme showed more mixed results (Humphrey, Lendrum and Wigelsworth 2010).

Seligman (2006) argues that we can change our responses to adversity. These ideas are often very useful not only to children with SEBCD but also to the adults who work with them, as it is sometimes possible to believe that their problems are insurmountable. Seligman suggests we examine our beliefs about something bad, for example a child who has lost his temper again. If we believe that he will never be able to change, the consequence might be that we stop helping him try. We can challenge negative or limiting thoughts by thinking about what evidence there is for this belief and what alternative explanations there are. We also need to think of the implications of this belief and how useful it is. A useful idea from solution-focused brief therapy (de Shazer and Dolan 2007) is looking for exceptions, so thinking of a time when the young person did not lose their temper may help reframe our thinking. Children and young people with SEBCD may have very negative feelings about themselves and their capabilities, so disputing their negative thoughts can change the negative feelings.

SELF-ESTEEM

Children and young people with SEBCD experience lots of failure, which can lead to low self-esteem. Low self-esteem seems to be linked with inappropriate behaviour, poor educational attainment and mental illness (Trzesniewski *et al.* 2006). Often children and young people would rather not attempt something new than face further failure. Increasing self-esteem is thought to be important, but it has to be considered carefully; a high self-worth which is just based on praise rather than on the development of useful skills could be counterproductive (Newman and Blackburn 2002).

Self-esteem is difficult to define, but it relates to a certain degree of competence and a positive view of oneself. Ideas about oneself develop from the opinions and reactions of others, so children and young people who are unable to interact well often receive very little positive feedback. Their self-esteem can be raised by positive feedback and information from others, thereby increasing self-worth. Sometimes the biggest challenge in raising self-esteem is finding positives to give genuine praise for, especially as there needs to be five times as many positive as negative comments for them to have any positive effect. However, praise can have negative effects if children or young people are told they are clever and then they face something they can't do; they may then suffer a lack of motivation. Therefore praising for effort is most effective (Cimpian *et al.* 2007).

In addition to praise for effort, it is important to offer opportunities to develop competence in areas such as communication, literacy and interaction skills, as suggested in this chapter. Problem-solving skills are also important. Problems can be resolved or worked on in some way, or even endured if necessary. Allowing, encouraging and supporting young people in their attempts to think and problem-solve increases self-esteem and enables them to become independent thinkers.

Positive interactions are likely to raise self-esteem, but the following strategies can also be effective in raising self-esteem:

- Accept the children although their behaviour may not be acceptable.

- Give positive feedback repeatedly and frequently; be concrete, specific, honest and accurate. Catch them doing things right, and remark on it. For example, 'You have worked hard at that'. Praise for who they are as well as what they do is also important. For example: 'That was kind. I've noticed you are often kind to him'.

- Earshotting: some young people find it difficult to accept praise directly, so let them overhear you saying something good about them.

- Set tasks you know they can accomplish, with effort, and then they know the praise is genuinely earned.

- Give them opportunities to record their own progress.

- Provide opportunities for them to help others, and take responsibility; then they have something to be proud of.

- Point out their strengths and give opportunities to use them.

- Encourage practice to achieve mastery in something they enjoy.

- Remind them of their achievements.

- Comment positively on their appearance.

- Comment on your own mistakes in a non-judgemental way, e.g. 'I know I can do that right if I try again', rather than 'I'm an idiot'.

- Try to deflect negative comments they or others may make about themselves, e.g. 'Rubbish is interesting' or 'Dung beetles love that'.

- Ask them to reflect on behaviour, take responsibility and understand the benefits of behaving well.

- Keep their optimism and confidence high by encouraging them to see any problems as temporary or restricted.

There seems to be a correlation between teacher and pupil self-esteem; adults with high self-esteem can raise that of their students (Lawrence 2006), so once again we need to look to ourselves.

PLAY

We have seen how play is important for symbolic development and provides opportunities to learn social, emotional, behavioural and communication skills. More than that, allowing rough and tumble play does seem to help children concentrate (Panksepp 2008), and offering play breaks seems to help children focus on tasks (Pellegrini 2006).

Furthermore, Panksepp also thinks that the way that the social brain grows is through enjoying play with others.

However, just providing toys or time to play may not be enough. If children and young people haven't had the opportunity or the encouragement to play, or if they are preoccupied with other things, they may need help to begin. Many children who have communication difficulties also have delays in the development of play skills.

Adults or young people may also think that play is only for children, but playing together is also a good way to develop positive relationships. Adults can help play skills develop by providing opportunities, modelling play, teaching games and by playing with children and young people. However, it's important not to lose sight of the fact that play should be fun, have no particular goals and be spontaneous and voluntary. Free play should be just that. When children are allowed, by adults who join in, to take the lead, their play is most advanced (Hurwitz 2002/03). Play can help cement adult–child relationships (Ginsburg 2007).

Encouraging imagining, especially how they could make things better (Novick 1998) can help young people see different possibilities and improve their creative thinking. Play can be an opportunity to act out daydreams and problem-solve. As a child begins to play symbolically, adults can give a 'running commentary' of their play; if the young person is not yet able to do this himself or herself, this can help develop both language and thinking skills. Suggesting verbal labels for the activities, feelings, needs or beliefs that the child expresses through play is a simple but effective technique. Group games also improve co-operation, especially if they are not competitive, if there is enough structure and if there are group rewards for working together. At about age three and a half, children start to play together and develop friendships, but some will need help to achieve this. Encouraging children to take specific roles in play may be helpful, so they learn different ways to interact. For example, LEGO therapy, where children are given specific roles such as engineer, supplier and builder, in order to help them work together, is currently being researched at the Cambridge Autism Research Unit (by Gomez de la Cuesta, Humphrey and Baron-Cohen).

SOCIAL COMMUNICATION SKILLS

We know that those who are resilient in difficult circumstances are likely to be those with good relationships though to adulthood (Collishaw *et al.* 2007). So helping children and young people with SEBCD develop the skills necessary to build positive relationships is very important. Social understanding skills, necessary for positive relationships, can be developed though play with peers, increasing co-operative social interaction and exposure to talk about feelings. However, these children and young people may need to learn basic social interaction skills before they can play with others. Problem behaviours often occur at play time or during unstructured activities, because the skills needed for joining in and negotiating roles are complex. Young people with SEBCD may well need support to learn these skills.

Adults may need to make explicit otherwise implicit rules, for example explaining why turn-taking and listening skills are important. If adults observe play and keep a record of who played with whom, what went well, whether there were any problems and why, this information can be used to help young people develop the skills they need. Tools such as the Social Play Record (White 2006) can be helpful for this. It is also possible to identify which sorts of prompts from adults are effective in encouraging children to interact (Girolametto, Weitzman and Greenberg 2005). For example, will the child respond to a prompt such as 'It's important to take turns', or do they need to be told, 'It's his turn now'? Do they need help to notice that someone is trying to join in, or to rephrase their attempt so it can be successful? Do adults need to suggest what to say, such as 'Say, can I have a go?'

A careful assessment of strengths and weaknesses in the 'use' of language is important in order to identify a baseline and guide intervention. There are various resources which are useful in assessing and teaching social communication skills, such as the Social Use of Language Programme (Rinaldi 1992) and Talkabout (Kelly 2003). Once an assessment is done, targets can be set in discussion with the young person involved. Whatever the skill or skills are, they have to be clearly defined and broken down. Targets need to be concrete, small and achievable. For example, good listening is generally defined as being still, looking at the speaker and being quiet – and then, of course, some sort of thinking about what has been said must take place. So a target about improving listening could include any or all of these.

More sophisticated skills such as the rules of conversation can also be learnt, and children and young people can research this by observing real conversations. 'Scripts' can be developed for starting a conversation or finding out about others. The rules grid may be a useful visual way to represent which sorts of interaction are appropriate in which situations (Devlin 2009). This could help a child or young person understand that 'Hello, mate' is OK as a greeting to a friend and possibly to a teacher you know well, but not to a stranger or a policeman.

Children and young people need to be provided with opportunities to practise new social communication skills in a safe environment, perhaps in a group, and then they need to be given opportunities to practise these in semi 'real' situations, where their attempts will be successful because those on the receiving end have been prompted to respond positively. After this, they can be encouraged to try their new skills in real situations and, of course, be praised when they succeed. Through the modelling of appropriate behaviours, practice in role-play and good accurate feedback (ideally using video), young people can change and develop their social communication skills (Reichow and Volkmar 2010).

MAKING FRIENDS

The value of friends cannot be underestimated. Subjective well-being seems to be linked to having strong social networks of family, friends and others (Johnson *et al.* 2010). Talking with friends helps children and young people develop their social, emotional, behavioural and communication skills. Friends also give emotional support, reduce isolation and provide extra resources for problem-solving, so it is worth persevering to develop friendships. This is not necessarily an easy task for young people with SEBCD; indeed it may be one of the most difficult things for them to achieve. Therefore trying to provide opportunities for young people with SEBCD to make friends is invaluable, as they may find it difficult to create opportunities for themselves.

Some children and young people with SEBCD may need to be taught how to make friends; for example, they may need to be given conversational starters, ideas about how to approach people and ways to introduce themselves. There also seem to be 'rules' of friendship which include:

- being reliable
- having fun
- sharing

- trying to resolve conflicts and forgive
- talking about yourself and asking questions of others
- expressing positive feelings about your friends.

'Circle of Friends' (Kalyva and Avramidis 2005) mobilises children and young people to provide a support network for their peers, whatever their difficulties, on the assumption that acceptance leads to change. It recognises the resources that young people have and their ability to be inclusive. It is easier to hear criticism or suggestions from peers than from people in authority, and this kind of approach can lead to more acceptable behaviour.

SOCIAL PROBLEM-SOLVING

A key friendship skill is being able to resolve problems. More fundamentally, the idea that problems can be solved is part of an active coping style which fosters resilience. The skills necessary for this are essentially the same as those outlined in 'solving problems with words' above. These are also known as 'conflict resolution strategies' and 'negotiation skills' and they are outlined below:

- Stop!
- Look and listen for clues.
- What is the problem? Gain an awareness of the whole situation: the perspectives, feelings and interests of those involved.
- What are the options for solving it?
- Consider the consequences of each of these.
- Work towards a win-win solution, where all parties are satisfied with the outcome.
- Decide what to do and implement the most effective.
- Reflect on your choice.

Many young people with SEBCD misunderstand social cues. They may assume that others are being hostile when they are not, or they may be so acutely aware of some cues they miss others, so learning to observe and think clearly about what is happening in an encounter can change the way they behave. Reflecting on unsuccessful attempts and thinking about another person's thoughts and feelings is also important in developing these skills (see Figure 6.5).

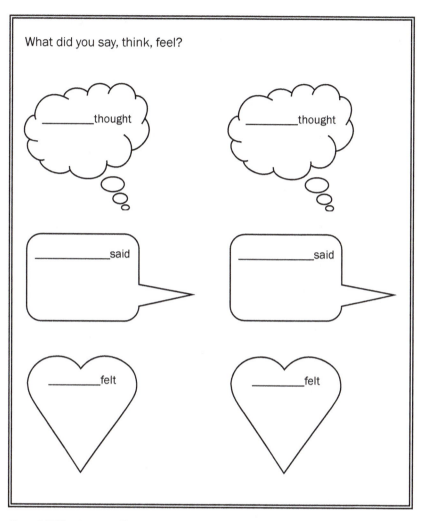

Figure 6.5 What happened?

Children with advanced social understanding are more co-operative; they can appreciate another point of view. These important skills can also be taught in everyday situations and they can improve the way a young person understands and relates to others. Adults can model the kind of 'self-talk' we use to think through difficult situations; 'Stay calm'; 'I wonder why he is so upset'; 'Let it go', etc. Seeing this kind of thinking 'in action' can validate it, and empower young people to try it for themselves. Conflict resolution training of this kind can be successful in the short term and in the longer term peer mediators can be effective (Blank *et al.* 2010). A vital factor in learning negotiation skills is children and young people interacting with adults who are willing to negotiate with them.

NARRATIVES

Some children need support to understand and tell stories. Limited narrative skills are common in children with SEBCD, and they lead to problems with understanding, remembering and retelling stories as well as with negotiation and problem-solving. Those who are able to construct a clear narrative about their lives and reflect on it are more likely to be securely attached, so making sure children have the language skills to do this is important.

One of the simplest ways to encourage an appreciation of narrative structure is to read stories to a child or young person, particularly if they have literacy difficulties, regardless of their age. Story tapes are useful for older children. Retelling stories with support, either in play or just through discussing what has been read (or seen on TV) can encourage an understanding of cause and effect. Additionally, retelling will lead to an understanding of the importance of the sequence of events, the emotions involved and the vocabulary used. Another useful strategy is starting a story and asking a young person to finish it either verbally or through play.

Before written narratives can develop, there has to be an appreciation and use of narrative structure in speech. Stories need a setting, information about characters, problems and solutions, as well as information about feelings. Without an appreciation of the structure of narratives and its most salient points, a child or young person can be overwhelmed with information when hearing a story. It is similarly difficult to begin on constructing a narrative without an appreciation of what the main points are. Once someone has an idea of what should be included in an account, and if they are given time to rehearse their ideas aloud and to develop a 'plan', then they can begin to construct written narratives. A narrative frame can be useful (Davies, Shanks and Davies 2004) to help children develop their narrative skills. An example of a narrative frame which can be customised with pictures is given in Figure 6.6.

Who?

Describe/draw them

Where?

When?

What happened?

How did they feel?

What did they do?

Figure 6.6 Narrative frame

MEMORY STRATEGIES

Given that many children with SEBCD have memory limitations, it is useful to teach strategies to overcome this. Several strategies have been found to be effective:

- making up a story or sentence which has the words to be remembered in it

- repeating what has to be remembered either out loud or silently

- visual imagery.

(Turley-Ames and Whitfield 2003)

Specific interventions
Prevention and early intervention

Early identification of communication difficulties and intervention is important because of the role that communication skills play in the development of emotional, social and cognitive skills. Similarly, early intervention for mental health difficulties seem to have long-term benefits (Hazell 2007). Interventions are more likely to be successful if they start early and go on longer, are intensive, directly affect children's lives, are broad in scope and if families are involved (Ramey and Ramey 1992). There is also evidence of the economic effectiveness of such early interventions (Reynolds *et al.* 2007). The Head Start programme in America targeted low income children by providing comprehensive services including preschool education; medical, dental, and mental health care; nutrition services; and efforts to help parents foster their child's development. It has been shown to have positive effects on the children's language skills and their interactions with their parents (US Department of Health and Human Services, Administration for Children and Families 2010). Programmes which support at-risk families, such as the Nurse–Family partnership programme currently being piloted in the UK, have also led to an improvement in the children's communication (Olds 2006).

If early intervention is to work for children with SEBCD, babies and children with attachment difficulties or behaviour problems should be screened for communication difficulties. Those who have problems with communication should also be screened for SEBD.

Support for parents

There is a great deal of research linking the quality of the parent–child relationship to a child's ability to learn and interact well (O'Connor and Scott 2007). The best outcomes occur when parents are authoritative; that is, they are warm, assertive and positive in their control, and they have high expectations as the child grows older. Parenting becomes more challenging when the child has communication problems and, of course, SEBD. Being a parent is also more difficult when one is living in stressful circumstances, perhaps in a poor, unsafe area.

It can be effective to provide support for parents and their families where necessary as in Head Start, the Nurse-Family partnerships and Sure Start in the UK. There are also various parenting programmes which can develop parenting skills. Some of these target the child's behaviour very effectively, for example a competence training programme for parents of socially disruptive children (Lauth, Otte and Heubeck 2009), Parent–Child Interaction Therapy and Triple P: Positive Parenting Program (Thomas and Zimmer-Gembeck 2007). The Incredible Years Programme (see www. incredibleyears.com) includes parent training which strengthens parenting competencies (monitoring, positive discipline, confidence) and fosters parents' involvement in children's school experiences. It has proved useful for many families and is effective for children with conduct problems and ADHD (Jones *et al.* 2007).

Other parenting programs target language; for example, the Hanen Early Language Parent Programme enables groups of parents to learn about communication difficulties and strategies they can use to help language development (see www.hanen.org). It has a positive effect on children's language growth (Girolametto *et al.* 1999). There are also programmes which include interventions to address both behaviour and language skills successfully for children with anti-social behaviour, such as the SPOKEs project (Hancock, Kaiser and Delaney 2002; Scott *et al.* 2010).

So, successful parenting interventions can lead to improved behaviour and communication in children because many of the skills parents need to help both language and behaviour develop in their children are similar.

Speech and language therapy

SLTs are familiar with typical language and communication development and can intervene when this does not occur. In addition to this, they have a role in helping others understand the communication skills gaps a child may have. SLTs also support caregivers and others to optimise their interactions with children and young people (Ahsam, Shepherd and Warren-Adamson 2006) and can suggest specific strategies to enhance language development. Furthermore, SLTs can work collaboratively to make interventions as accessible as possible for children and young people with SEBCD.

Increased understanding of communication problems can help make interactions more positive. Often it is assumed that a child or young person does understand but is not being co-operative, so a speech and language therapy assessment of what they can and cannot understand, and what resources they have to express themselves, can be very useful. Once adults understand that behaviours might be at least in part due to communication difficulties, their view of the child may change. A young person may be seen as unco-operative, but they may have such difficulty understanding language that they avoid conversations whenever they can. Another child who can't say 'I don't like that, stop it', may bite instead; once people interacting with the child understand this, they can respond more appropriately.

Research has shown that speech and language therapy can be effective (Law, Garrett and Nye 2003), but that short-term interventions are less effective (Law 2000). While there is evidence for the effectiveness of speech and language therapy, there is still only a small amount of evidence to draw on (Cirrin and Gillam 2008), so there is an urgent need for more research. Nonetheless, the inclusion of SLTs as part of a multidisciplinary team in Sure Start is improving the quality of provision for vulnerable young children (Ofsted 2009). Speech and language therapy can also be effective for problems with the use of language (Adams and Lloyd 2007), to help children develop their narrative skills (Davies *et al.* 2004), story comprehension (Joffe, Cain and Maric 2007), vocabulary (Best 2005; Parsons, Law and Gascoigne 2005) and grammar (Ebbels 2007).

School-based approaches, including those working in groups (Boyle *et al.* 2009; Joffe 2006) have facilitated changes in the approaches used by teaching staff and in children's communication skills (Boyle and Forbes 2007; Roulstone, Owen and French 2005). Well-trained and supported teaching assistants or speech and language therapy assistants can also effectively improve children's communication skills (McCartney, Ellis and Boyle 2009; Mecrow, Beckwith and Klee 2010).

Moreover, there is evidence that speech and language therapy can be effective with children and young people with SEBD. Law and Sivyer

(2003) showed that SLT was able to improve the narrative, vocabulary and social communication skills of a group of children with SEBD. Similarly Heneker (2005) was able to develop the communication skills of ten children in a pupil referral unit (PRU). Stringer's (2006) work led to a significant improvement in the communication skills of adolescents with SEBD. It seems that speech and language therapy can also improve behavioural skills (Law and Plunkett 2009).

Ritzman and Sanger (2007) showed that the language pathology (SLT in the UK) service for children with SEBD was valued and that it impacted on social adjustment, academic performance and behaviour. The same seems to be true in prisons. 'I have to admit that in all the years I have been looking at prisons and the treatment of offenders, I have never found anything so capable of doing so much for so many people at so little cost as the work that speech and language therapists carry out' (Ramsbotham 2006).

Mostly, the SLT support for children with SEBCD who need to develop their communication skills is the same as for any child or young person with communication problems. However, their SEBD also needs to be understood and accommodated by the SLT. Some slightly different approaches might be useful to enhance positive interactions which can be hard to establish. Non-directive speech and language therapy has grown out of theories of play therapy (Cogher 1999), essentially providing a young person with a running commentary (in appropriate language for them) as they play without suggesting how they play or what they do. The benefits of this are that the young person is focusing on something while hearing the verbal labels for it, and the lack of direction encourages them to be more exploratory. It can be a useful tool in working with children and young people with SEBD, who may not co-operate with more directive activities.

Gallagher (1999, p.12) suggests that SLTs need to help children with SEBCD in the following ways:

- Teach communicative alternatives to unacceptable behaviours.
- Build event-based script knowledge for socially or emotionally difficult situations.
- Manipulate antecedent behaviours to increase opportunities to practise positive communicative behaviours.
- Reward socially positive communication behaviours.
- Develop broader and more varied emotional vocabularies.

SLTs can also work to help children learn the skills to make friends, peer group entry, conflict resolutions and inclusion social skills (Ostrov and Godleski 2007).

Unfortunately, even if all children with SEBCD were identified, there are very few SLTs working with children who have SEBD. However, this is slowly changing as schools and foster care agencies employ SLTs, and as a greater awareness of the positive role SLTs can play in mental health services develops (Law and Garrett 2004).

Foster care

Foster carers do a remarkable job with abused, neglected and traumatised young people. If small children are taken into care in their first year of life and live with carers who are sensitive to their needs, they are able to form positive attachments despite what went before (Dozier *et al.* 2001).

Mental health interventions

There are many effective interventions for young people with mental health difficulties and their families (Kazdin and Weisz 2009; Roth and Fonagy 2006). For example, infant–parent psychotherapy (IPP), and psychoeducational parenting intervention (PPI) have both been shown to be effective at increasing secure attachment in abusive families (Cicchetti, Rogosch and Toth 2006). Play therapy is also valuable with children (Bratton *et al.* 2005). It is particularly useful for those who are unable, for various reasons, to put their feelings into words.

The family is an interactive and interdependent system, and it is often a mistake to focus on the individual who has the 'symptoms', because they are part of a system that influences their behaviour and that behaviour serves a function for the family. For example, families who have children with very difficult behaviour tend to have defensive communications, blame each other more and tend not to support one another. Therefore the goal of family therapy is to improve communication and mutual support by helping them see the 'problem' from other points of view. Multisytemic therapy, which considers other systems of which the child is part, as well as the family, has been shown to be effective in improving behaviour in adolescents (Carr 2009).

Data from meta-analyses of randomised controlled trials of CBT (there has been a lot of research into CBT as it lends itself to quantitative research methodologies in a way that other psychotherapies do not) suggest that it is most useful for children and adolescents with generalised anxiety disorder, depression, obsessive compulsive disorder and PTSD (Butler *et al.* 2006). There is a useful leaflet for young people about CBT on the Royal College of Psychiatrists website (Royal College of Psychiatrists 2008).

Solution-focused brief therapy is, as the title suggests, a focus on solutions rather than problems. It assumes that everyone has the resources they need to succeed, and it tries to focus on these rather than on problems. So, instead of the problem, young people are encouraged to think about what they'd like to be doing instead, and do it. This approach has proved effective (Kim 2008) and useful in schools (Franklin, Kelly and Kim 2008).

Given this plethora of effective treatments, it can be difficult to decide which approach is going to be appropriate for which child. For those who have been abused and neglected, CBT may have more of an effect on behaviour, play therapy more on social functioning, and individual and family therapy on distress (Hetzel-Riggin, Brausch and Montgomery 2007). However there is also evidence that the 'therapeutic alliance' or the relationship is more important than the type of treatment (Green 2006). Client centred therapy is based on unconditional positive regard, genuineness and empathy. So the therapeutic alliance offers safety, boundaries, consistency, authentic responses, trust and spontaneity that result in containment, in the same way as a secure attachment does.

However, how can young people access a 'talking therapy' if they have difficulty with communication (Cohen 2001)? Children with communication difficulties certainly have difficulty with abstract language such as metaphor (Norbury 2005) and often with simpler concepts such as who and why. Stacey (1995) considers ways in which family therapists can enable language-impaired children to access the language of therapy. She suggests using concrete explanations, using analogy rather than metaphor and rephrasing or acting out questions. She considers this to be vital in order to include their ideas and not marginalise them in therapy. Psychotherapy has been shown to have a positive effect on language development for some children with mild communication problems (Russell, Greenwald and Shirk 1991), probably because the children experience individual attention and responsiveness that clarifies and expands on what they are trying to communicate.

Nonetheless, we are not sure which interventions might work for children with SEBCD. It is still likely that they might receive parallel approaches to SEBD and communication problems, so there is still considerable scope for more 'joined up' approaches. A step forward would be more communication assessments of children and young people with mental health difficulties, which could inform those delivering the approach so they are able to modify it where necessary.

In school

There is little evidence to guide teachers as to how to best support children with SEBD in mainstream schools, let alone those with SEBCD. It may be that students with SEBCD are more sensitive to any negative aspects of schooling, as learning is always an emotional experience and they often have fewer resources to draw on in order to be tolerant (Cooper 1996). In learning, one is exposing one's ignorance, which is not possible without feeling secure in the situation where learning occurs. However, there is evidence that some schools do well with pupils with complex needs, so it is worth considering how they do that, as well as considering how schools provide specific interventions useful for those with SEBD and those with communication problems.

Some schools are able to engage disaffected young people (Ofsted 2008b). These are schools where the staff are committed to help the pupils succeed and they make this clear to the pupils and their families. One aspect of these schools is robust monitoring of academic, personal and social progress, and close collaboration with other services to ensure that pupils who were at risk were identified and supported.

So for pupils with SEBCD, this involves the identification of their communication problems, opportunities to learn social and emotional skills, as well as appropriately differentiated teacher talk, and tasks. This is reflected in recent behaviour guidance. 'It has long been recognised that securing the constructive engagement of pupils involves the planning of learning experiences that are relevant, engaging and appropriately differentiated' (Steer 2009, point 4.17).

Positive relationships are particularly important, as there is evidence that negative teacher–child relationships are related to children's later behaviour problems (Brendgen *et al.* 2007). For a learning experience to be fruitful there needs to be a sharing for information, experience, feelings and attention and the communication of a feeling of competence (Russell, Amod and Rosenthal 2008).

Schools also have a role in helping pupils develop appropriate behaviour. Powell and Tod (2004) in a review of the literature concluded that the following could promote positive behaviour:

- promoting learning as something valuable and meaningful in itself rather than just a way of achieving marks or targets
- using mixed-ability groupings and facilitative teaching approaches
- promoting on-task verbal interaction between pupils
- working in partnership with pupils in goal-setting so that a shared understanding can be established in relation to anticipating and addressing barriers to learning
- discouraging competitive classroom contexts and encouraging positive inter-personal relationships.

A review of the literature (Evans *et al.* 2003) found that rewarding good behaviour had positive effects, as did teaching self-monitoring, and that putting children in rows increased on-task behaviour. Modifications can also be made to the classroom environment to make it easier for students with SEBCD. Audet and Tankersley (1999) outline simple ways to alter the physical arrangement of the class, transitions between activities and classes, time structure and instructional demands in order to make it easier for such students. Visual representations of rules and expectations as well as the timetable can be helpful. In addition, adults using appropriate language levels are, of course, vital.

The behaviour policies of a school and adult interactions to improve behaviour should also take into account that pupils may not understand language well, be able to explain themselves clearly or have the required social communication skills.

As regards more specific interventions, with the advent of programmes such as SEAL (the Social and Emotional Aspects of Learning), there has been an acknowledgement that emotions exist in school, and that they have an effect on learning. Such interventions seem to work best when:

- they are integrated across the curriculum
- school staff take responsibility for effective emotional learning
- school staff have been transformed by addressing their own mental health needs and feel trained and supported before addressing the needs of students

- there are warm relationships including respectful and empathic compassionate concern
- there is positive behaviour management
- there are opportunities to learn from peers including through mentoring, mediation, conflict resolution and buddying
- there are opportunities for student voice with students and staff empowered to make real choices, and with appropriate levels of genuine decision-making and responsibility
- there is parental involvement.

(Nind and Weare 2009)

It is also important to make sure the language used in teaching such lessons is accessible and that pupils are given enough appropriate opportunities to learn the relevant emotion vocabulary.

'Nurture groups' (Boxall and Lucas 2010) started as an early years intervention for children with SEBD based on attachment theory. They are small groups which provide a bridge between home and school.

The six principles of nurture (the 'nurture group network') are:

- Learning is understood developmentally.
- The classroom offers a safe base.
- Nurturing is important for the development of self-esteem.
- Language is a vital means of communication.
- All behaviour is communication.
- Transitions are significant in the lives of children.
- Transitions are important in the lives of children and young people.

(The Nurture Group Network undated)

Nurture groups now exist in various forms. Sometimes children access them part-time, and they are also developing in secondary schools. They seem to be an effective way to support children and young people with SEBD (Cooper and Whitebread 2007), and they contribute to a positive school ethos. Such settings are also very useful for children with SEBCD.

The UK Resilience Programme is based on cognitive behaviour principles carried out in schools. Early evaluations have shown positive effects on children's anxiety and depression symptoms (Challen *et al.* 2009).

Clearly children with SEBCD also need specific teaching to develop their communication skills. In the UK the importance of speaking and listening as a basis of all learning, especially literacy, has often been underestimated. However, in one study, children with reading comprehension difficulties made more progress when taught oral language skills than when they worked on reading comprehension alone (Clarke *et al.* 2010). However, speaking and listening as part of the curriculum has come to the fore recently and these skills should be measured in school (using APP – Department for Children, Schools and Families 2010a).

Allowing opportunities for interaction and discussion and encouraging small group work can enable less verbal students to say more, feel more able to take risks with thinking, and to learn necessary social communication skills. Individual conversation activities can also help improve children's language skills in preschool (McCabe *et al.* 2009). Providing activities which encourage students to ask questions, take decisions and problem-solve also enables them to become active, independent learners. Collaborative philosophical enquiry for children (or 'real' discussion) has been shown to improve children's language and thinking skills (Topping and Trickey 2007).

However, there are still lessons where the adults dominate the conversations, which are not fertile ground for learning in general or language learning and which further disadvantage those with communication difficulties. Consider how tiring focusing on structured language-based activities is for someone with communication difficulties (see Rinaldi 1996). Providing support for pupils during unstructured time such as playtime and co-operative learning activities may be necessary to make them positive situations.

There is also more of a focus now on helping pupils understand how they learn and what helps them. For example, pupils with auditory processing difficulties may benefit from visual or kinaesthetic support materials. Davis and Florian (2004) conducted a review of the evidence for teaching approaches for children with SEN; the scarcity of research is such that they could only identify 'promising approaches'. These included teaching approaches that adopt additional (visual) reinforcement strategies to supplement verbal instruction. The popular idea of learning styles, for example being a predominantly visual or auditory learner, is not necessarily helpful. The idea of focusing on one style is not reinforced by research and the approach is under-theorised (Coffield *et al.* 2004). Different learning styles may be required for different tasks and it is important that pupils are exposed to different ways of learning and see their relative merits (Coffield 2005). It is most important for children to know how they learn best and what kind of strategies support their weaker modalities; this is particularly important for pupils with SEBCD, especially where their communication difficulties are not always recognised.

In order to support children with communication problems, it is necessary to modify the lesson structure and content, its delivery and possibly the classroom. Programmes such as I CAN's Talk programmes provide structures for various professionals to work together to achieve this, making schools as communication friendly as possible.

Strategies which help pupils with SEBCD in school include:

- opportunities to develop communication and emotional skills in lessons
- clear instructions, rules and routines supported by pictures and symbols
- a behaviour policy which takes into account possible SEBCD
- complex vocabulary explained and specific opportunities to learn core and across curriculum vocabulary
- frequent opportunities to check understanding
- narrative structures for writing and speaking, for example presentations, persuasion, etc.
- help to make links between tasks and outcomes and how things link together, e.g. 'We are learning this because....'

In ISP schools (those run by the Integrated Services Programme – an independent, not-for-profit child care organisation which mostly works with children and young people in foster care), teachers and SLTs work together to help children and young people develop their communication, emotional and thinking skills, but this is relatively rare.

Improving interactions through video

Many useful approaches for SEBCD centre on improving interaction and a helpful tool to support this is video (Anderson 2006). Video interaction guidance (VIG) is a technique which is based on attachment theory and which identifies positive interactions. It has been used in various contexts, such as with parents and children, teachers and pupils and adults whose working relationships are problematic.

Those taking part in VIG decide on a helping question: What is the problem they want to solve? Often it is about the child's communication or behaviour, perhaps, 'What do I do to help him talk?' or 'How can I stop him doing that?' or 'How do I get them to work together?' The video interaction guider takes a short (10–15 minute) video in a naturalistic setting. This video is edited to show a few sections where the interaction was successful in terms of the helping question. To help in this process the contact principles, indications of attunement (Biemans 1990), are referred to. Figure 6.7 shows how these principles could apply to children with SEBCD.

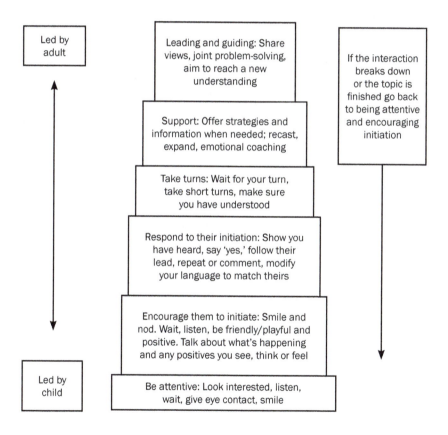

Figure 6.7 How VIG principles could apply to children with SEBCD

Through this process, people see their strengths and build on them. They have themselves as a positive role model. The process is non-directive and supportive, and people are guided to see their strengths.

VIG works by increasing self-awareness and reflection; it increases self-esteem, attuned responses and activates clients to solve their own problems. VIG is a useful tool for training professionals to increase responsive interactions and language stimulation in daycare settings (Fukkink and Tavecchio 2007). It can also help teachers develop their interaction for the benefit of young children (Fukkink and Tavecchio 2010). Fukkink (2008) undertook a meta analysis of VIG and found the effects were that parents were more skilled at interacting with their children, experienced fewer problems and gained more pleasure from them. The effect was greater when the intervention was short (less than seven feedbacks) and when focused on specific behavioural elements. VIG, sometimes known as video home training, has also been shown to be more effective than other parent-based interventions in having positive, long-term effects on children's language development (van Balkom *et al.* 2010). So, overall, VIG is a very promising intervention for children with SEBCD and those who interact with them.

Research and evaluation

There is little research about which are the most effective interventions for children with SEBCD, although we have plenty of good ideas to be getting on with. After all, 'Not everything that can be counted counts, and not everything that counts can be counted' (Einstein). Nonetheless it is important for interventions for SEBCD to evaluate the effect they have on social, emotional, behaviour and communication skills (Law and Plunkett 2009). This can present a challenge because of the complexity of the issues involved; it is difficult to know what to measure and how to measure it.

The lack of evidence is also due to a lack of funding for research, especially into communication problems in children and young people. Despite communication problems being ten times as common as autism, for example, much less research funding is available. This inequity needs to change.

Conclusion

Much can be done to help young people with SEBCD, but in order for this to occur some major changes are necessary:

- Children and young people with SEBD should be screened for communication difficulties.

- Also, young people with communication difficulties should be screened for SEBD.

- There needs to be a recognition that children with SEBCD are not all the same, so a range of interventions and services are necessary.

- Early and ongoing intervention for children with SEBCD is important.

- Children with SEBCD need comprehensive and integrated service delivery regardless of what is seen as their 'primary' difficulty.

- SLTs should be part of the team around the child or young person who has SEBCD.

- Interventions for children and young people with SEBCD and mental health difficulties should be audited for their language demands so they can be more effective.

- In times of limited resources, we have to consider whether those who get services are those who need them most, those who can benefit from them most, or those who have the most vocal advocates.

Helping young people with SEBCD develop their communication skills is likely to contribute to their social capital and therefore their ability to live fulfilling lives and contribute to society. Sadly the reverse is also true.

Appendix 1

Indicators List for Identifying Communication Difficulties

Young person's name:

Year group/age:

Completed by:

Date:

Understanding language	Tick if applicable
Has difficulties following long or complex instructions E.g. 'You need to read the chapter and then identify the key ideas which you then need to write about, explaining why they are important'	
Has better understanding in a 1:1 situation than in a group Knows and understands what is said in 1:1 yet in a whole class or group situation is confused	
Watches and copies others when instructions are given	
Has difficulties recalling information or putting it into the right sequence Unable to remember and recount last week's episode of a soap on TV	
Tends to take things literally When told 'I'll be back in a minute', expects the person to literally come back to them in 60 seconds	
Gives an inappropriate response to abstract language 'Keep your hair on' results in their looking confused or asking about their hair	
Repeats what you say rather than responding appropriately 'What have you been reading?' 'I've been reading'	

Has difficulties understanding implied meaning 'I wouldn't take my shoes off now' meaning 'Don't take your shoes off': interpreted as you talking about yourself	
Is slow to learn new routines Finds it difficult to learn new ideas and language especially in sequence	
Doesn't listen when people talk too much or use complex language May lose focus or get frustrated	

Form	*Tick if applicable*
Speaks too quickly Others cannot follow what has been said	
Is not easy to understand When talking about spies, says 'pies'; some words not intelligible	
Says the same word differently at different times Hospital: hotpital, hosital	
Stammers Hesitates, repeats sounds/words, gets stuck	
Has difficulties with prepositions and tenses Misuses or misses out; on, under, over, ran, running	
Has difficulties using sentences with conjunctions Including 'and', 'because', 'so', or uses these words too much	
May take a long time to organise words into a sentence Pauses for a long time before responding or stops mid sentence, searching for a word	
Misses out words or puts them in the wrong order 'Last night football played park' for 'Last night I played football in the park'	
Has difficulties giving specific answers or explanations 'I dunno, it's kind of, something that's, well you know…'	
Has difficulties recalling and sequencing events and ideas appropriately Finds it difficult to remember or tell a story, even a simple one	

Content	Tick if applicable
Has limited vocabulary Uses same core vocabulary which could lead to excessive swearing	
Finds it hard to express emotions verbally Can't explain how they are feeling or why	
Uses fluent, clear speech which doesn't seem to mean much 'Came over to that place and did that you know'	
Has trouble learning new words Names of people and objects	
Cannot provide significant information to listeners Difficult for the listener to understand what they are trying to say	
Uses made-up words which are almost appropriate 'Window worker man'	
Overuses 'meaningless' words Thingy, whatever, that	

COPYRIGHT © I CAN 2009. ADAPTED FROM WORK BY
MELANIE CROSS AND ANGELA SLOAN IN CROSS (2004).

Use	Tick if applicable
Has difficulties with eye contact or personal space Doesn't make eye contact or gets too close to others	
Interrupts inappropriately Not aware when it is and isn't appropriate to say something	
Avoids situations which require words Social situations, reading out loud or presenting to others	
Is unable to vary language with the situation Uses the same language with peers, teachers and unfamiliar adults	
Has problems recognising and responding to non-verbal cues Doesn't notice if someone is sad, puzzled, etc.	
Attracts attention in inappropriate ways or without words Annoys others, fiddles with things, or sits quietly and does their own thing	
In conversation, moves from topic to topic for no obvious reason or finds it difficult to change the subject 'Do I need to type this up, so can I go and talk to Sam, I like your earrings'	
Has difficulties taking turns in conversation Always monopolises the conversation or doesn't understand when someone has a different view and changes the focus	
Doesn't ask questions or start a conversation Sits quietly and waits for others to initiate verbal communication	
Doesn't say if they can't understand Will continue doing what they are doing even if it isn't what was asked for	
Has difficulty persuading and negotiating May give up or get frustrated	
Has difficulty solving problems with words May use no verbal means	

Appendix 2

Strategies for Supporting Communication Problems

Difficulties understanding language	
The child or young person:	**Tips to help:**
Has difficulties following long or complex instructions 'You need to read the chapter and then identify the key ideas which you then need to write about, explaining why they are important'	• Repeat and rephrase where necessary. • Slow your speech and insert more pauses. • Use shorter sentences. • Emphasise key words. • Use visual cues to support key words. • Encourage to ask or signal when they don't understand. • Encourage them to summarise what you've just said.
Has better understanding in a 1:1 situation than in a group Knows and understands what is said in 1:1 yet in a whole class or group situation is confused	• Use child or young person's name at start of instructions to focus them. • Reduce background distractions. • Make sure you are facing the child or young person when giving information. • Say, 'Everyone needs to listen to this'.

Watches and copies others when instructions are given	• Cue them in when instructions or changes of topic are imminent.
	• Provide visual cues to support understanding.
	• Scaffold ideas by linking new concepts to familiar ones.
	• Ask them to focus on you and tell you if it doesn't make sense.
	• Help them recognise when they don't understand.
Has difficulties recalling information or putting it into the right sequence Unable to remember and recount last week's episode of a soap on TV	• Use visual cues such as pictures, objects and diagrams to help recall information.
	• Use visual timetables to sequence events.
	• Use mind maps to capture ideas.
	• Narrative frames, e.g. who, where, when, what happened, etc.
	• Prompt with cues such as first, then, last.
	• Ask them to give feedback about which parts they did and didn't follow.
	• Encourage them to say what they have to remember 'in their head'.
Tends to take things literally When told 'I'll be back in a minute', expects the person to literally come back to them in 60 seconds	• Check understanding of and explicitly teach idioms such as 'get a grip'.
	• Think about the language that you use and whether literal interpretations are possible.
	• Simplify your language and explain if you use abstract or idiomatic language.
Gives an inappropriate response to abstract language 'Keep your hair on' results in their looking confused or asking about their hair	• Prepare child or young person for new abstract language by pre-teaching.
	• Explain the different possible meanings.
	• Prompt to ask for clarification.

Repeats what you say rather than responding appropriately 'What have you been reading?' 'I've been reading'	• Check that the child or young person understands the language that you have been using. • Offer a simpler version of what you just said. • Use visual prompts to support understanding.
Has difficulties understanding implied meaning 'I wouldn't take my shoes off now' meaning 'Don't take your shoes off': interpreted as you talking about yourself	• Use specific and concrete language. • Use visual cues including gestures to support spoken language. • Show the child or young person what you mean. • Discuss how people use indirect language.
Is slow to learn new routines Finds it difficult to learn new ideas and language especially in sequence	• Repeat previous information. • Use visual support (writing and speaking frames as well as pictures and symbols) to aid recall and spoken language. • Give plenty of time for the child or young person to think things through before responding.
Doesn't listen when people talk too much or use complex language May lose focus or get frustrated	• Simplify your language and pause. • Give the young person time to contribute. • Give opportunities to ask for clarification.

Form: Structure of their communication	
The child or young person:	**Tips to help:**
Speaks too quickly Others cannot follow what has been said	• Record the child or young person talking and see if they recognise when they speak quickly. • Agree on a way of signalling to the child or young person when they are starting to speed up. • Make sure they are not rushed or feeling rushed.
Is not easy to understand When talking about spies, says 'pies'; some words not intelligible	• Do not correct; instead give the right model of spoken language, e.g. 'Oh, there was a spy!' • Respond to what they are trying to say rather than how. • Sometimes you may have to say (kindly) that you can't understand and perhaps there's another way to explain it.
Says the same word differently at different times Hospital: hotpital, hosital	• Do not correct; instead give the right model of spoken language, e.g. 'She was in hospital?' • Support words with visual cues such as objects and pictures.
Stammers Hesitates, repeats sounds/words, gets stuck	• Seek advice from local speech and language therapy team. • Be calm and patient yourself. • Give the child or young person time to think before responding. • Allow the child or young person time to finish what they are saying rather than finishing their sentence for them. • Do not put pressure on them to speak or read aloud.
Has difficulties with prepositions and tenses Misuses or misses out; on, under, over, ran, running	• Respond to them including a grammatically correct version of what they said. So if they say 'I brang it', say 'great, you brought it'. • Use visual information to support grammatical structures, e.g. gesture, pictures. • Colour code different words — works best if a whole school approach. • Underline particular grammatical structures to emphasise them.

Has difficulties using sentences with conjunctions Including 'and', 'because', 'so', or uses these words too much	• Provide sentence frames with examples of how to use 'and', 'because' and 'so'. • Stress these words in your own explanations. • Repeat their versions including these words as a model.
May take a long time to organise words into a sentence Pauses for a long time before responding or stops mid sentence, searching for a word	• Allow time to think. • Use visual cues including objects, pictures, diagrams, mind maps and personal dictionaries to support spoken language. • Listen and show your interest by maintaining eye contact and using their name.
Misses out words or puts them in the wrong order 'Last night football played park' for 'Last night I played football in the park'	• Give the child or young person the right language model without criticising what they have said. • Colour code words so that they know which words they need and teach how to sequence them.
Has difficulties giving specific answers or explanations 'I dunno, it's kind of, something that's, well you know...'	• Ask questions with forced alternatives: 'Do you need to read the information or go and ask someone?' • Offer choices of vocabulary for them to select from. • Use visually supporting information to help the child or young person recall details, link words and ideas. • Give them time.
Has difficulties recalling and sequencing events and ideas appropriately Finds it difficult to remember or tell a story, even a simple one	• Check the child or young person understands how to sequence; what is first, next/in the middle and last/at the end. • Use story frames with start, middle, end and pictures or questions to support thinking. • Mind map ideas then use ideas in a story frame.

Content	
The child or young person:	**Tips to help:**
Has limited vocabulary Uses same core vocabulary which could lead to excessive swearing	• Use visual strategies to develop vocabulary, e.g. word cards, pictures, real objects, symbols, mind maps and personal dictionaries all involving combinations of words, pictures, drawing and colours. • Reinforce new vocabulary in different contexts; perhaps have 'words of the week' to focus on in different contexts. • Decide on which are the key words per topic and provide many opportunities to learn them. • Help students learn new words by discussing the sounds they start with, how many syllables they have, what they rhyme with, what they look like, their function, where you'd find them, what categories they belong to, their opposites, what they make you think of. Also use drama and gesture where possible. Silliness helps: e.g. 'me and her' could help a student remember 'meander' if it was illustrated by two women meandering beside a river. • Help them link new words with what they already know.
Finds it hard to express emotions verbally Can't explain how they are feeling or why	• Use pictures of different facial expressions to explore the vocabulary of emotions and how the child or young person experiences the emotion. • Discuss how tone of voice and posture give clues to emotions. • Discuss the emotions of characters in stories or history. • Encourage the child or young person to think about and discuss how stories, TV, films, events and discoveries make them feel. • Discuss how people manage their emotions. • Use SEAL materials across the curriculum.

Uses fluent, clear speech which doesn't seem to mean much 'Came over to that place and did that you know'	• Develop vocabulary skills through experiences, visually supporting information and repetition. • Refer to narrative frame: 'This sounds interesting but I don't know where it happened.' • Teach structure for narrative including beginning, middle and end.
Has trouble learning new words Names of people and objects	• Limit the number of new words to be learnt and give explicit opportunities (as above); choose words which will be most useful: either those for things which interest the child or young person or those which will be of most value. • Provide clear, consistent definitions of abstract words as well as examples of how they can be used. • Repeat words with visual support in different contexts. Start with the real thing, then small models, then photographs or symbols. • Use personal dictionaries. • Provide plenty of opportunities for repetition and revision.
Cannot provide significant information to listeners Difficult for the listener to understand what they are trying to say	• Use symbols and visual cues to trigger the child or young person to respond to certain questions: who, what, where, when, etc. • Give clear instructions which are written down and supported by visual cues to guide the child or young person's responses. • Repeat what you think the child or young person said so they can tell you if you are right.
Uses made-up words which are almost appropriate 'Window worker man'	• Use mind maps and concept maps to enable the student to link thoughts, ideas and words to a topic. • Use personal whiteboards on which the child or young person can note down words or images which help them recall words. • Model appropriate language; for example 'Yes, it's a window cleaner' in response to 'window worker man'.
Overuses 'meaningless' words Thingy, whatever, that	• Use visual cues including objects, pictures, diagrams and photos to remind and prompt use of other vocabulary. • Use forced alternative questions to elicit specific responses; for example 'Was it a boy or a girl?'

Use	
The child or young person:	**Tips to help:**
Has difficulties with eye contact or personal space Doesn't make eye contact or gets too close to others	• Explain the effect on the listener when these rules are broken and perhaps explore through role play. • Encourage children or young people to signal that they are listening by making brief eye contact. • Ask them to look at the person they are speaking to. • Suggest they look at others' faces to see signs of discomfort to help them judge the right distance.
Interrupts inappropriately Not aware when it is and isn't appropriate to say something	• Praise good listening skills. • Encourage to wait for a gap or a clear signal from the speaker. • Teach useful phrases such as 'Can I just say...', 'Sorry to interrupt, but...' and 'Sorry, you go ahead...' • Make class/home rules about who can speak and when explicit, e.g. Is it always hand up? Or wait for a gap?
Avoids situations which require words Social situations, reading out loud or presenting to others	• Try to understand why, build language skills, help with preparation, and structure and develop confidence in smaller groups as necessary.
Is unable to vary language with the situation Uses the same language with peers, teachers and unfamiliar adults	• Explain about different codes and how its useful to have more than one as it widens your choices/options in the future. • Discuss the effects of saying the wrong thing to the wrong person. • Point out what you feel is rude and why. • Model the language you'd like to hear.
Has problems recognising and responding to non-verbal cues Doesn't notice if someone is sad, puzzled, etc.	• Point out these non-verbal cues using video/TV/mirrors. • Link these cues to people's feelings and subsequent actions.

Attracts attention in inappropriate ways or without words Annoys others, fiddles with things, or sits quietly and does their own thing	• Make expectations for getting attention clear; put your hand up, ask for help, etc. • Check that the quiet child is focused on the task and understands what they have been asked to do as well as how to complete the task.
In conversation, moves from topic to topic for no obvious reason or finds it difficult to change the subject 'Do I need to type this up, so can I go and talk to Sam, I like your earrings'	• Explain: 'You've changed topics so I can't follow. What was the first question?' • Be explicit: 'We're only talking about volcanoes now.' • 'That's interesting, but now we're onto...'
Has difficulties taking turns in conversation Always monopolises the conversation or doesn't understand when someone has a different view and changes the focus	• Use a bar chart to track how much of the conversation each person has. Is it equally shared? • Use social stories to explain how turn-taking works and why it is important to listen to other people's views. • Use video to help them see what they do when it works.
Doesn't ask questions or start a conversation Sits quietly and waits for others to initiate verbal communication	• Pause, listen, look at the student and smile. • Explain how important it is to have ideas from everyone. • Perhaps it is easier for them to initiate in some situations; use those. • Help them prepare what they want to say in a non-threatening situation before contributing to a larger group. • Check they have the necessary language skills. • Work in pairs or small groups. • Discuss the value of everyone's contribution. • Offer conversation starters: 'My view is...' • Don't put pressure on them to speak. • Comment on what they've achieved rather than asking questions.

Doesn't say if they can't understand Will continue doing what they are doing even if it isn't what was asked for	• Make sure they know when they don't understand, ask them to repeat what they think they have to do. • Teach clarification strategies, e.g. 'Can you say that again please?' • Encourage asking when they don't understand; give opportunities and praise when they do. • Teach questions to use: 'What does X mean?' or 'Can you break that up for me, please?' • Respond positively to anyone asking for clarification: 'Thanks. It's useful to know if it doesn't make sense.'
Has difficulty persuading and negotiating May give up or get frustrated	• The language and emotional skills necessary may need to be explicitly taught. • Offer opportunities to practise where they can succeed.
Has difficulty solving problems with words May use no verbal means	• The language and emotional skills necessary may need to be explicitly taught. • Offer opportunities to practise where they can succeed.

Glossary of Abbreviations

ADHD	Attention deficit hyperactivity disorder
Afasic	Association For All Speech-Impaired Children
APP	Assessing Pupils' Progress
ASD	Autism spectrum disorder
BESD	Behavioural, emotional and social difficulties
BMA	British Medical Association
CBT	Cognitive behaviour therapy
CDS	Child directed speech
DCD	Developmental co-ordination disorder (dyspraxia)
DCSF	Department for Children, Schools and Families
DH	Department of Health
DSM	Diagnostic and Statistical Manual of Mental Disorders
ERRNI	Expression, Reception and Recall of Narrative Instrument
GCSE	General Certificate of Secondary Education
ICD	International Classification of Diseases
ICF	International Classification of Functioning
IPP	Infant–parent psychotherapy
IQ	Intelligence Quotient
ISP	Integrated Services Programme
MHD	Mental health difficulty
NEET	Not in education, employment or training
NICHD	National Institute of Child Health and Human Development
NVIQ	Non-verbal Intelligence Quotient
PATHS	Promoting Alternative Thinking Strategies
PPI	Psychoeducational parenting intervention
PTSD	Post-traumatic stress disorder
SEAL	Social and Emotional Aspects of Learning
SEBCD	Social, emotional, behavioural and communication difficulties

SEBD Social, emotional and behavioural difficulties

SEN   Special educational needs

SES   Socio-economic status

SLI   Specific language impairment

SLT   Speech and language therapist

UK   United Kingdom

US   United States

VIG   Video interaction guidance

WHO World Health Organization

References

Achenbach, T. M. (1991) *Manual for the Child Behaviour Checklist 4–18*. Burlington, VT: University of Vermont Press.

Achilles G. M., Mclaughlin M. J. and Croninger R. G. (2007) 'Socio-cultural correlates of disciplinary exclusion among students with emotional, behavioral and learning disabilities in the SEELS national dataset.' *Journal of Emotional and Behavioral Disorders 15*, 1, 33–45.

Ackerman, B. (1982) 'On comprehending idioms: Do children get the picture?' *Journal of Experimental Psychology 33*, 439–54.

Adams, C., Coke, R., Crutchley, A., Hesketh, A. and Reeves, D. (2001) *Assessment of Comprehension and Expression 6–11 (yrs)*. London: NFER–NELSON.

Adams, C. and Lloyd, J. (2007) 'The effects of speech and language therapy intervention on children with pragmatic language impairments in mainstream school.' *British Journal of Special Education 34*, 4, 226–233.

Adamson-Macedo, E. N., Patel, R. and Sallah, D. K. (2009) 'An independent psychometric evaluation of a speech and language tool for two-year-old children from a sure start trailblazer site in the West Midlands.' *Child Language Teaching and Therapy 25*, 2, 191–214.

Afasic (1991) *Checklists, age 4–10*. Available at www.afasicengland.org.uk/publications/resources-for-professionals, accessed on 22 January 2011.

Ahsam, S., Shepherd, J. and Warren-Adamson, C. (2006) 'Working with pre-school practitioners to improve interactions.' *Child Language Teaching and Therapy 22*, 2, 197–217.

Ainsworth, M. D. S., Blehar, M., Waters, E. and Wall, S. (1978) *Patterns of Attachment: A Psychological Study of the Strange Situation*. Hillsdale, NJ: Erlbaum.

American Psychiatric Association (1994) *Diagnostic and Statistical Manual of Mental Disorders, 4th edition* (DSM-IV). Washington, DC: American Psychiatric Association.

Anderson, C. (2006) 'Early communication strategies: Using video analysis to support teachers working with preverbal pupils.' *British Journal of Special Education 33*, 3, 114–120.

Antoniazzi, D., Snow, P. and Dickson-Swift, V. (2010) 'Teacher identification of children at risk for language impairment in the first year of school.' *International Journal of Speech Language Pathology 12*, 3, 244–252.

Archibald, L. M. and Gathercole, S. E. (2006) 'Short-term and working memory in specific language impairment.' *International Journal of Communication Disorders 41*, 6, 675–693.

Arnold, E. M., Goldston, D. B., Walsh, A. K., Reboussin, B. A. *et al.* (2005) 'Severity of emotional and behavioral problems among poor and typical readers.' *Journal of Abnormal Child Psychology 33*, 2, 205.

Audet, L. R. and Tankersley, M. (1999) 'Implications of Communication and Behavioural Disorders for Classroom Management: Collaborative Intervention Techniques.' In D. Rogers-Adkinson and P. Griffith (eds) *Communication Disorders and Children with Psychiatric and Behavioural Disorders.* San Diego, CA, and London: Singular Publishing Group Inc.

Audit, L. and Ripich, D. N. (1994) 'Psychiatric Disorders and Discourse Problems.' In N. D. Ripich and N. A. Craighead (eds) *School Discourse Problems.* San Diego, CA: Singular Publishing Group Inc.

Bandstra, E. S., Morrow, C. E., Vogel, A. L., Fifer, R. C. *et al.* (2002) 'Longitudinal influence of prenatal cocaine exposure on child language functioning.' *Neurotoxicology and Teratology* 24, 3, 297–308.

Baron-Cohen, S. (2009) 'Autism: The empathizing-systemizing (E-S) theory.' *Annals of the New York Academy of Sciences 1156*, 68–80.

Baron-Cohen, S. and Belmonte, M. K. (2005) 'Autism: A window onto the development of the social and the analytic brain.' *Annual Review of Neuroscience 28*, 109–126.

Bastian, V., Burns, N. and Nettelbeck, T. (2005) 'Emotional intelligence predicts life skills, but not as well as personality and cognitive abilities.' *Personality and Individual Differences 39*, 1135–1145.

Bates, E., Thal, D. and Janowsky, J. S. (1992) 'Early Language Development and Its Neural Correlates.' In S. J. Segalowitz and I. Rapin (eds) *Handbook of Neuropsychology 7*, 69–110. Amsterdam: Elsevier.

Beals, D. E., DeTemple, J. M. and Dickinson, D. K. (1994) 'Talking and Listening that Support Early Literacy Development of Children from Low-Income Families.' In D. K. Dickinson (ed.) *Bridges to Literacy: Children, Families, and Schools.* Cambridge, MA: Basil Blackwell.

Beaver, K. M., Delisi, M., Vaughn, M. G., Wright, M. G. and Boutwell, B. B. (2008) 'The relationship between self-control and language: Evidence of a shared pathway.' *Criminology* 46, 4, 939–970.

Bedford, J. (2008) *Social Communication Profile.* Vancouver, B.C.: Black Sheep Press.

Beeghly, M. and Cicchetti, D. (1994) 'Child maltreatment, attachment, and the self-system: Emergence of an internal state lexicon in toddlers at high social risk.' *Development and Psychopathology 6*, 5–30.

Behne, T., Carpenter, M., Call, J. and Tomasello, M. (2005) 'Unwilling versus unable: Infants' understanding of intentional action.' *Developmental Psychology 41*, 2, 328–337.

Beitchman, J. H. and Cohen, N. J. (eds) (1996) *Language, Learning, and Behavior Disorders: Developmental, Biological, and Clinical Perspectives.* New York: Cambridge University Press.

Benasich, A. A., Choudhury, N., Friedman, J. T., Realpe Bonilla, T., Chojnowska, C. and Gou, Z. (2006) 'Infants as a prelinguistic model for language learning impairments: Predicting from event-related potentials to behavior.' *Neuropsychologia 44*, 3, 396–411.

Benner, G. J., Mattison, G. J., Nelson, R. and Ralston, R. N. C. (2009) 'Types of language disorders in students classified as ED: Prevalence and association with learning disabilities and psychopathology. *Education and Treatment of Children 32*, 4.

Benner, G. J., Nelson, R. and Epstein, M. H. (2002) 'Language skills of children with EBD: A literature review.' *Journal of Emotional and Behavioural Disorders 10*, 1, 43–59.

Bennett, L. P. (2005) 'A broad conceptual framework for the development and management of young people's behavioural difficulties.' *Educational and Child Psychology 22*, 3, 6–16.

Bercow, J. (2008) *Bercow Review of Services for Children and Young People (0–19) with Speech, Language and Communication Needs (2008)*. Reference no.: DCSF-00632-2008. Available at www.dcsf.gov.uk/bercowreview, accessed on 22 January 2011.

Berquez, A. (2009) 'Continuing professional development for stammering: Does it make a difference?' Presentation at Royal College of Speech and Language Therapists scientific conference, *Partners in Progress: Spreading the Word*, 17 March 2009.

Berridge, D. (2007) 'Theory and explanation in child welfare: Education and looked-after children.' *Child and Family Social Work 12*, 1–10.

Best, W. (2005) 'Investigation of a new intervention for children with word-finding problems.' *International Journal of Language Communication Disorders 40*, 3, 79–318.

Biemans, H. (1990) 'Video Home Training: Theory Method and Organization of SPIN.' In J. Kool (ed.) *International Seminar for Innovative Institutions*. Ryswyck: Ministry of Welfare Health and Culture.

Bishop, D. V. M. (1994) 'Is specific language impairment a valid diagnostic category? Genetic and psycholinguistic evidence.' *Philosophical Transactions of the Royal Society B: Biological Sciences 346*, 105–111.

Bishop, D. V. M. (1998) 'Development of the Children's Communication Checklist (CCC): A method for assessing qualitative aspects of communicative impairment in children.' *Journal Child Psychology Psychiatry 39*, 6, 879–91.

Bishop, D. V. M. (2004) *Expression, Reception and Recall of Narrative Instrument (ERRNI)*. London: Pearson Assessment.

Bishop, D. V. M. (2010) *The common childhood disorders that have been left out in the cold*. Available at www.guardian.co.uk/science/2010/dec/01/sli-autism-childhood-developmental-disorders, accessed on 22 January 2011.

Bishop, D. V. M. and McDonald, D. (2009) 'Identifying language impairment in children: Combining language test scores with parental report.' *International Journal Language Communication Disorders 44*, 5.

Bishop, D. V. M. and Norbury, C. F. (2002) 'Exploring the borderlands of autistic disorder and specific language impairment: A study using standardised diagnostic instruments.' *Journal of Child Psychology and Psychiatry 43*, 917–929.

Bishop, D. V. M., Whitehouse, A. J .O. and Sharpe, M. (2009) *Communication Checklist: Self Report (CC-SR)*. London: Pearson.

Black, D. S., Milam J. and Sussman, S. (2009) 'Sitting-meditation interventions among youth: A review of treatment efficacy.' *Pediatrics 124*, 3, 532–541.

Blager, F. B. (1979) 'The effect of intervention on speech and language of abused children.' *Child Abuse and Neglect 5*, 991–996.

Blanden, J. (2006) 'Bucking the trend: What enables those who are disadvantaged in childhood to succeed later in life?' *Working Paper No. 31*. London: Department for Work and Pensions.

Blank, L., Baxter, S., Goyder, E., Naylor, P. B. *et al.* (2010) 'Promoting well-being by changing behaviour: A systematic review and narrative synthesis of the effectiveness of whole secondary school behavioural interventions.' *Mental Health Review Journal 5*, 2.

Blanton, D. J. and Dagenais, P. A. (2007) 'Comparison of language skills of adjudicated and non-adjudicated adolescent males and females.' *Language, Speech, and Hearing Services in Schools 38*, 309–314.

Bleses, D., Vach, W. and Lum, J. A. G. (2010) 'Linguistic profiles in language delayed three-year-old children: Evidence for gender specific differences.' Presentation at Child Language Seminar, City University, London.

Bloom. L. and Beckwith, R. (1989) 'Talking with feeling: Integrating affective and linguistic expression in early language development.' *Cognition and Emotion* 3, 313–342.

BMA Board of Science (2006) *Child and Adolescent Mental Health: A Guide for Healthcare Professionals.* London: British Medical Association. Available at www.bma.org.uk/images/ ChildAdolescentMentalHealth_tcm41-20748.pdf, accessed on 5 July 2011.

Bor, W., Brennan, P. A., William, G. M., Najman, J. M. and O'Callaghan, M. (2003) 'A mother's attitude towards her infant and child behaviour five years later.' *Australian and New Zealand Journal of Psychiatry* 37, 748–55.

Botting, N. and Conti-Ramsden, G. (2000) 'Social and behavioural difficulties in children with language impairment.' *Child Language Teaching and Therapy* 16, 2, 105–120.

Bowlby, J. (1969) *Attachment and Loss* (Vol. 1 Attachment). London: Hogarth.

Boxall, M. and Lucas, S. (2010) *Nurture Groups in Schools: Principles and Practice.* London: Paul Chapman.

Boyle, J. E. and Forbes, J. A. (2007) 'A randomised controlled trial and economic evaluation of direct versus indirect and individual versus group modes of speech and language therapy for children with primary language impairment.' *Health Technology Assessment* 11, 25, 1–158.

Boyle, J. M., McCartney, E., O'Hare, A. and Forbes, J. (2009) 'Direct versus indirect and individual versus group modes of language therapy for children with primary language impairment: Principal outcomes from a randomised controlled trial and economic evaluation.' *International Journal of Language and Communication Disorders* 44, 6, 826–84.

Bratton, S. C., Ray, D., Jones, L. and Rhine, T. (2005) 'The efficacy of play therapy with children: A meta-analytic review of treatment outcomes.' *Professional Psychology: Research and Practice* 36, 4.

Brendgen, M., Wanner, B., Vitaro, F., Bukowski, W. M. and Tremblay, R. E. (2007) 'Verbal abuse by the teacher during childhood and academic, behavioral, and emotional adjustment in young adulthood.' *Journal of Educational Psychology* 99, 26–38.

Brinton, B., Spackman, M. P., Fujiki, M. and Ricks, J. (2007) 'What should Chris say? The ability of children with specific language impairment to recognize the need to dissemble emotions in social situations.' *Journal of Speech Language and Hearing Research* 50, 3, 798–811.

Brophy, M. and Dunn, J. (2002) 'What did mummy say? Dyadic interactions between young "hard to manage" children and their mothers.' *Journal of Abnormal Child Psychology* 30, 2.

Brown, J. R. and Donelan-McCall, N. (1993) 'Talk with your mother or your siblings? developmental changes in early family conversations about feelings.' *Child Development* 63, 336–349.

Brownlie, E. B., Beitchman, J. H., Escobar, M., Young, A. *et al.* (2004) 'Early language impairment and young adult delinquent and aggressive behaviour.' *Journal of Abnormal Child Psychology* 32, 4, 453–67.

Brownlie, E. B., Jabbar, A., Beitchman, J., Vida, R. and Atkinson, L. (2007) 'Language impairment and sexual assault of girls and women: Findings from a community sample.' *Journal of Abnormal Child Psychology* 35, 4, 618–626.

Bruce, B., Thernlund, G. and Nettelbladt, U. (2006) 'ADHD and language impairment: A study of the parent questionnaire FTF (Five to Fifteen).' *European Child and Adolescent Psychiatry 15*, 152–60.

Bryan, K. (2004) 'Preliminary study of the prevalence of speech and language difficulties in young offenders.' *International Journal of Language and Communication Disorders 39*, 3, 391–400.

Bryan, K., Freer, J. and Furlong, C. (2007) 'Language and communication difficulties in juvenile offenders.' *International Journal of Language and Communication Disorders 42*, 5, 505–520.

Burchinalab, M., Howesc, C., Piantad, R., Bryanta, D. *et al.* (2008) 'Predicting child outcomes at the end of kindergarten from the quality of pre-kindergarten teacher–child interactions and instruction.' *Applied Developmental Science 12*, 3, 140–153.

Burgess, J. and Bransby, G. (1990) 'An evaluation of the speech and language skills of children with emotional and behavioural problems.' *College of Speech Therapy Bulletin 453*, 2–3.

Buschmann, A., Jooss, B., Rupp, A., Dockter, S. *et al.* (2008) 'Children with developmental language delay at 24 months of age: Results of a diagnostic work-up.' *Developmental Medicine and Child Neurology 50*, 3, 223–229.

Butler, A. C., Chapman, J. E., Forman, E. M. and Beck, A. T. (2006) 'The empirical status of cognitive-behavioral therapy: A review of meta-analyses.' *Clinical Psychology Review 26*, 1, 17–31.

Butler, I. and Williamson, H. (1994) *Children Speak, Children Trauma and Social work.* Harlow: Longman Publishing.

Camilleri, B. and Law, J. (2007) 'Assessing children referred to speech and language therapy: Static and dynamic assessment of receptive vocabulary.' *International Journal of Speech-Language Pathology 9*, 4, 312–322.

Campbell, T. F., Dollaghan, C., Needleman, H. and Janosky, J. (1997) 'Reducing bias in language assessment: Processing dependent measures.' *Journal of Speech, Language and Hearing Research 40*, 519–529.

Campbell, T. F., Dollaghan, C.A., Rockett, H. E., Paradise, J. L. *et al.* (2003) 'Risk factors for speech delay of unknown origin in 3-year-old children.' *Child Development 74*, 2, 346–357.

Cardy, J. E., Tannock, R., Johnson, A. M. and Johnson, C. J. (2010) 'The contribution of processing impairments to SLI: Insights from attention-deficit/hyperactivity disorder.' *Journal of Communication Disorders 43*, 2, 77–91.

Carlson, S. M. (2009) 'Social origins of executive function development.' *New Directions for Child and Adolescent Development 123*, 87–98.

Carr, A. (2009) 'The effectiveness of family therapy and systemic interventions for child-focused problems.' *Journal of Family Therapy 31*, 1, 3–45.

Catts, H. W., Adlof, S. M., Hogan, T. P. and Weismer, S. E. (2005) 'Are specific language impairment and dyslexia distinct disorders?' *Journal of Speech, Language, and Hearing Research 48*, 6, 1378–1396.

Caulfield, M. B. (1989) 'Communication difficulty: A model of the relation of language delay and behaviour problems.' *Society for Research in Child Development Abstracts 7*, 212.

Challen, A., Noden, P., West, A. and Machin, S. (2009) UK Resilience Programme Evaluation Research Report Interim Report DCSF-RR094.

Champagne, S. and Cronk, C. (1998) 'Le mutisme sélectif étudié à travers l'expérience d'un échantillon d'orthophonistes québécois. Fréquences.' *Canadian Association of Speech Language Pathologist Journal, Quebec 10,* 4, 23–26.

Chiat, S. and Roy, P. (2007) 'The preschool repetition test: An evaluation of performance in typically developing and clinically referred children.' *Journal of Speech, Language and Hearing Research 50,* 429–443.

Chiat, S. and Roy, P. (2008) 'Early phonological and socio-cognitive skills as predictors of later language and social communication outcomes.' *Journal of Child Psychology and Psychiatry 49,* 6, 635–645.

Cicchetti, D., Rogosch, F. A. and Toth, S. L. (2006) 'Fostering secure attachment in infants in maltreating families through preventive interventions.' *Development and Psychopathology 18,* 623–649.

Cimpian, A., Arce, H., Markman, E. M. and Dweck, C. S. (2007) 'Subtle linguistic cues impact children's motivation.' *Psychological Science 18,* 314–316.

Cirrin, F. M. and Gillam, R. B. (2008) 'Language intervention practices for school-aged children with spoken language disorders: A systematic review.' *Language Speech and Hearing Services in Schools 39,* 110, 137.

Clark, A., O'Hare, A., Watson, J. and Cohen, W. (2007) 'Severe receptive language disorder in childhood – familial aspects and long-term outcomes: Results from a Scottish study.' *Archive of Disorders in Childhood 92,* 7, 614–619.

Clarke, P. J., Snowling, M. J., Truelove, E. and Hulme, C. (2010) 'Ameliorating children's reading-comprehension difficulties a randomized controlled trial.' *Psychological Science 21,* 8, 1106–1116.

Clegg, J., Hollis, C., Mawhood, L. and Rutter, M. (2005) 'Developmental language disorders – a follow-up in later adult life. Cognitive, language and psychosocial outcomes.' *Journal of Child Psychology and Psychiatry 46,* 2, 128–149.

Clegg, J., Stackhouse, J., Finch, K., Murphy, C. and Nicholls, S. (2009) 'Language abilities of secondary age pupils at risk of school exclusion: A preliminary report.' *Child Language Teaching and Therapy 25,* 1.

Coffield, F. (2005) *Learning Styles: Help or Hindrance?* NSIN Research Matters, Institute of Education, University of London.

Coffield, F., Moseley, D., Hall, E. and Eccleston, K. (2004) *Learning Styles and Pedagogy in Post-16 Learning: A Systematic and Critical Review.* London: Learning and Skills Research Centre.

Cogher, L. (1999) 'The use of non-directive play in speech and language therapy.' *Child Language Teaching and Therapy 15,* 1, 7–15.

Cohan, S. L., Chavira, D. A., Shipon-Blum, E., Hitchcock, C., Roesch, S. C. and Stein, M. B. (2008) 'Refining the classification of children with selective mutism: A latent profile analysis.' *Journal of Clinical Child and Adolescent Psychology 37,* 4.

Cohen, J. S. and Mendez, J. L. (2009) 'Emotion regulation, language ability and the stability of preschool children's peer play behaviour.' *Early Education and Development 20,* 6, 1016–1037.

Cohen, N. J. (2001) *Language Impairment and Psychopathology in Infants, Children and Adolescents.* Thousand Oaks, California: Sage Publications.

Cohen, N. J. (2003) 'Overlap of communication impairments and social-emotional problems in infants.' *IMPrint 37,* 19–21.

Cohen, N. J., Barwick, M. A., Horodezky, N. B., Vallance, D. D. and Im, N. (1998) 'Language, achievement, and cognitive processing in psychiatrically disturbed children with previously identified and unsuspected language impairments.' *Journal of Child Psychology and Psychiatry 39*, 6, 865–877.

Cohen, N. J., Davine, M., Hordezky, M. A., Lipsett, L. and Isaacson, B. A. (1993) 'Unsuspected language impairments in psychiatrically disturbed children: Prevalence and language and behavioural characteristics.' *Journal of the American Academy of Child and Adolescent Psychiatry 32*, 595–603.

Cohen, N. J. and Lipsett, L. (1991) 'Recognised and unrecognised language impairment in psychologically disturbed children. Child symptomatology maternal depression and family dysfunction.' *Canadian Journal of Behavioural Science 23*, 3, 376–389.

Collishaw, S., Pickles, A., Messer, J., Rutter, M., Shearer, C. and Maughan, B. (2007) 'Resilience to adult psychopathology following childhood maltreatment: Evidence from a community sample.' *Child Abuse and Neglect 31*, 211–229.

Conti-Ramsden, G. (2008) 'Heterogeneity of Specific Language Impairment in Adolescent Outcomes.' In C. Frazier Norbury, J. B. Tomblin and D. V. N. Bishop (eds) *Understanding Developmental Language Disorders, from Theory to Practice.* Abingdon: Psychology Press.

Conti-Ramsden, G. and Botting, N. (2004) 'Social difficulties and victimization in children with SLI at 11 years of age.' *Journal of Speech, Language, and Hearing Research 47*, 145–161.

Conti-Ramsden, G., Durkin, K., Simkin, Z. and Knox, E. (2009) 'Specific language impairment and school outcomes 1; Identifying and explaining variability at the end of compulsory education.' *International Journal of Communication Disorders 44*, 1, 15–35.

Conti-Ramsden, G., Simkin, Z. and Botting, N. (2006) 'The prevalence of autistic spectrum disorders in adolescents with a history of specific language impairment (SLI).' *Journal of Child Psychology and Psychiatry 47*, 621–628.

Cooper, P. (1996) 'The Inner Life of Children with Emotional and Behavioural Difficulties.' In V. P. Varma (ed.) *The Inner Life of Children with Special Needs.* London: Whurr Publishers.

Cooper, P. and Whitebread, D. (2007) 'The effectiveness of nurture groups on student progress: Evidence from a national research study.' *Emotional and Behavioural Difficulties 12*, 3, 171–190.

Crittenden, P. M. (1995) 'Attachment and Psychopathology.' In S. Goldberg, R. Muir and J. Kerr (eds) *Attachment Theory: Social, Developmental and Clinical Perspectives.* Hillsdale, NJ: The Analytic Press.

Cross, M. (1999) 'Lost for words.' *Child and Family Social Work 42*, 249–257.

Cross, M. (2001) 'Undetected communication problems in children who are looked after by the local authority.' Unpublished MPhil thesis, Cardiff University.

Cross, M. (2004) *Children with Emotional and Behavioural Difficulties and Communication Problems: There is Always a Reason, 1st edition.* London: Jessica Kingsley Publishers.

Cross, M., Blake, P., Tunbridge, N. and Gill, T. (2001) 'Collaborative working to promote the communication skills of a 14-year-old student with emotional, behavioural, learning and language difficulties.' *Child Language Teaching and Therapy 17*, 3, 227–246.

Crystal, D., Garman, M. and Fletcher, P. (1976) *The Grammatical Analysis of Language Disability: A Procedure for Assessment and Remediation*, 2nd edn. London: Cole and Whurr.

Dahl, R. E. and Spear, L. P. (eds) (2001) 'Adolescent brain development: Vulnerabilities and opportunities.' *Annals of the New York Academy of Sciences 1021*.

Dallos, R. and Draper R. (2010) *An Introduction to Family Therapy: Systemic Theory and Practice.* Berkshire: Open University Press.

Davies, P., Shanks, B. and Davies, K. (2004) 'Improving narrative skills in young children with delayed language development.' *Educational Review 56,* 3, 271–286.

Davis, P. and Florian, L. (2004) *Teaching Strategies and Approaches for Pupils with Special Educational Needs: A Scoping Study. Research Report 516.* London: DfES Publications.

De Bellis, M. D. (2003) 'The Neurobiology of Posttraumatic Stress Disorder Across the Life Cycle.' In D. Moore and J. Jefferson (eds) *The Handbook of Medical Psychiatry.* London: Elsevier.

De Bellis, M. D., Keshavan, M. S., Frustaci, K., Shifflett, H. *et al.* (2002a) 'Superior temporal gyrus volumes in maltreated children and adolescents with PTSD.' *Biological Psychiatry 51,* 544–552.

De Bellis, M. D., Keshavan, M. S., Shifflett, H., Iyengar, S. *et al.* (2002b) 'Brain structures in pediatric maltreatment-related PTSD: A socio-demographically matched study.' *Biological Psychiatry 52,* 11, 1066–1078.

De Rosnay, M. and Harris, P. L. (2002) 'Individual differences in children's understanding of emotion: The roles of attachment and language.' *Attachment and Human Development 4,* 1, 39–54.

de Shazer, S. and Dolan, Y. (2007) *More Than Miracles: The State of the Art of Solution-focused Brief Therapy.* Binghamton, NY: The Haworth Press.

Denham, S. A., Renwick, S. M. and Holt, R. W. (2008) 'Working and playing together: Prediction of preschool social emotional competence from mother–child interaction.' *Child Development 16,* 2, 242–249.

Department for Children, Schools and Families (2008a) *Revised Guidance on the Education of Children and Young People with Behavioural, Emotional and Social Difficulties (BESD).* Available at www.teachernet.gov.uk/wholeschool/behaviour/schooldisciplinepupilbehaviourpolicies/besdguidance/ accessed on 24 January 2011.

Department for Children, Schools and Families (2008b) *Targeted Mental Health in Schools Project: Using the Evidence to Inform Your Approach: A Practical Guide for Headteachers and Commissioners, DCSF-00784-2008.* Available at www.education.gov.uk/publications/standard/publicationdetail/page1/DCSF-00784-2008, accessed on 9 June 2011.

Department for Children, Schools and Families (2008c) *Inclusion Development Programme.* Available at http://webarchive.nationalarchives.gov.uk/20110202093118/http://nationalstrategies.standards.dcsf.gov.uk/search/inclusion/results/nav:46335, accessed on 12 July 2011.

Department for Children, Schools and Families (2009) *Lamb Inquiry: Special Educational Needs and Parental Confidence.* Available at www.education.gov.uk/publications/standard/publicationdetail/page1/DCSF-01143-2009, accessed on 9 June 2011.

Department for Children, Schools and Families (2010a) *Assessing Pupils' Progress in English at Key Stage 3.* Available at https://nationalstrategies.standards.dcsf.gov.uk/node/303361?uc=force_uj, accessed on 22 January 2011.

Department for Children, Schools and Families (2010b) *The Use of Force to Control or Restrain Pupils Guidance for Schools in England.* Available at www.teachernet.gov.uk/docbank/index.cfm?id=14800, accessed on 22 January 2011.

Department for Education and Skills (2001) *Special Educational Needs Code of Practice*. Available at www.teachernet.gov.uk/_doc/3724/SENCodeofPractice.pdf, accessed on 22 January 2011.

Department for Education and Skills (2003) *National Curriculum Attainment Target 1: English 1, Speaking and Listening*. Available at http://curriculum.qcda.gov.uk/key-stages-1-and-2/subjects/english/attainmenttargets/index.aspx, accessed on 22 January 2011.

Desforges, C. and Abouchaar, A. (2003) *The Impact of Parental Involvement, Parental Support and Family Education on Pupil Achievement and Adjustment: A Literature Review*. Research Report 43. London: DfES Publications.

Devescovi, A. and Caselli, M. C. (2007) 'Sentence repetition as a measure of early grammatical development in Italian.' *International Journal of Language and Communication Disorders 42*, 187–208.

Devlin, N. (2009) 'The rules grid: Helping children with social communication and interaction needs manage social complexity.' *Educational Psychology in Practice 25*, 4, 327–338.

Dewart, H. and Summers, S. (1995) *The Pragmatics Profile of Everyday Communication Skills in Children*. Windsor: NfrNelson.

DH (2004) *National Service Framework for Children, Young People and Maternity Services*. London: DH. Available at www.dh.gov.uk/en/Publicationsandstatistics/Publications/PublicationsPolicyAndGuidance/DH_4089100, accessed on 6 July 2011.

Dionne, G., Tremblay, R., Boivin, M., Laplante, D. and Pérusse, D. (2003) 'Physical aggression and expressive vocabulary in 19-month-old twins.' *Developmental Psychology 39*, 2, 261–273.

Dixon, W. E. and Smith, P. H. (2000) 'Links between early temperament and language acquisition.' *Merril-Palmer Quarterly 46*, 3, 417–40.

Dockrell, J., Lindsay, G., Palikara, O. and Cullen, M. (2007) *Raising the Achievements of Children and Young People with Specific Speech and Language Difficulties and Other Special Educational Needs through School to Work and College*. DfES Research Report RR837. London: University of London, Institute of Education.

Doidge, N. (2008) *The Brain That Changes Itself*. London: Penguin.

Domes, G., Heinrichs, M., Michel, A., Berger., C. and Herpertz, S. C. (2007) 'Oxytocin improves "mind-reading" in humans.' *Biological Psychiatry 61*, 6, 731–733.

Dominey, P. F. and Dodane, C. (2004) 'Indeterminacy in language acquisition: The role of child-directed speech and joint attention.' *Journal of Neurolinguistics 17*, 2–3, 121–145.

Donno, R., Parker, G., Gilmour, J. and Skuse, D. H. (2010) "Social communication deficits in disruptive primary-school children.' *The British Journal of Psychiatry 196*, 282–289.

Dowrick, P. W., Kim-Rupnow, W. S. and Power, T. J. (2006) 'Video feedforward for reading.' *Journal of Special Education 39*, 4, 197–204.

Dozier, M., Stovall, K. C., Albus, K. E. and Bates, B. (2001) 'Attachments for infants in foster care: The role of caregiver state of mind.' *Child Development 75*, 2, 1467–1477.

Duchan, J. (1989) 'Evaluating adults' talk to children: Assessing adult attunement.' *Seminars in Speech and Language 10*, 17–27.

Durand, V. M. and Merges, E. (2001) 'A Contemporary Behavior Analytic Intervention for Problem Behaviors.' *Focus on Autism and Other Developmental Disabilities 16*, 2, 110–119.

Durham, R. E., Farkas, G., Scheffner, Hammer, C., Tomblin, J. B. and Catts, H. W. (2007) 'Kindergarten oral language skill: A key variable in the intergenerational transmission of socio-economic status.' *Research in Social Stratification and Mobility 25*, 4, 294–305.

Durkin, K. and Conti-Ramsden, G. (2010) 'Young people with specific language impairment: A review of social and emotional functioning in adolescence.' *Child Language Teaching and Therapy 26*, 2, 105–121.

Dyck, M. and Piek, J. (2010) 'How to distinguish normal from disordered children with poor language or motor skills.' *International Journal Language and Communication Disorders 45*, 3, 336–344.

Ealing Quality Indicators (2010) *Supporting All Children's Communication Development.* Available at www.childrenscentres.org.uk/eyfs_resources.asp?q=printme, accessed on 22 January 2011.

Ebbels, S. (2007) 'Teaching grammar to school-aged children with specific language impairment using shape coding.' *Child Language Teaching and Therapy 23*, 1, 67–93.

Eisenberg, N., Smith, C. L., Sadovsky, A. and Spinrad, T. L. (2004) 'Effortful Control: Relations with Emotion Regulation, Adjustment, and Socialization in Childhood.' In R. F. Baumeister and K. D. Vohs (eds) *Handbook of Self-regulation: Research, Theory and Applications.* New York: Guilford Press.

Elgen, I., Bruaroy, S. and Laegreid, L. M. (2006) 'Lack of recognition and complexity of foetal alcohol neuro-impairments.' *Acta Pædiatrica 96*, 2, 237–241.

Elliott, N. (in preparation) 'An investigation into the communication skills of long-term unemployed young men.' Interim results from a PhD study.

Emerson, E. and Hatton, C. (2007) 'Mental health of children and adolescents with intellectual disabilities in Britain.' *The British Journal of Psychiatry 191*, 493–499.

Ensor, R. and Hughes, C. (2005) 'More than talk: Relations between emotion understanding and positive behaviour in toddlers.' *British Journal of Developmental Psychology 23*, 3, 343–363.

Evangelou, M., Brooks, G., Smith, S. and Jennings, D. (2005) *The Birth to School Study: A Longitudinal Evaluation of the Peers Early Education Partnership (PEEP) 1998–2005.* London: DfES Publications.

Evans, G. W., Maxwell, L. and Hart, B. (1999) 'Parental language and verbal responsiveness to children in crowded homes.' *Developmental Psychology 35*, 1020–1023.

Evans J., Harden, A., Thomas, J. and Benefield, P. (2003) 'Support for pupils with emotional and behavioural difficulties (EBD) in mainstream primary classrooms: A systematic review of the effectiveness of interventions.' Research evidence in education library. London: University of London, Institute of Education, EPPI-Centre, Social Science Research Unit.

Fabes, R. A., Eisenberg, N., Hanish, L. D. and Spinrad, T. L. (2001) 'Preschoolers spontaneous emotion vocabulary: Relations to likability.' *Early Education and Development 12*, 11–27.

Farkas, J. and Beron, K. (2004) 'The detailed age trajectory of oral vocabulary knowledge: Differences by class and race.' *Social Science Research 33*, 464–497.

Farmer, M., Robertson, B., Kenny, C. and Siitarinen, J. (2008) 'Language and the development of self-understanding in children with communication difficulties.' *Educational and Child Psychology 24*, 4.

Faupel, A. (2003) (ed.) *Emotional Literacy: Assessment and Intervention.* Southampton Psychology Service, London: NferNelson Publishing.

Feinstein, L., Duckworth, K. and Sabates, R. (2004) *A Model of the Inter-generational Transmission of Educational Success.* The Centre for Research on the Wider Benefits of Learning, Institute of Education.

Feltis, B. B., Powell, M. B., Snow, P. C. and Hughes-Scholes, C. H. (2010) 'An examination of the association between interviewer question type and story-grammar detail in child witness interviews about abuse.' *Child Abuse and Neglect 34*, 6, 407–413.

Fenson, L., Dale, P. S., Reznick, J. S., Bates, E., Thal, D. J. and Pethicke, J. (1994) 'Variability in early communicative development.' *Monographs of the Society for Research in Child Development 59*, 1–173.

Fey, M. E., Long, S. H. and Cleave, P. (1994) 'Reconsideration of IQ criteria in the definition of specific language impairment.' In R. V. Watkins and M. Rice (eds) *Specific Language Impairments in Children 4*, 161–178. Baltimore, MD: Brookes.

Fonagy, P. (2003) 'Editorial: Towards a developmental understanding of violence.' *The British Journal of Psychiatry 183*, 190–192. Available at http://bjp.rcpsych.org/cgi/content/full/183/3/190, accessed on 22 January 2011.

Fonagy, P. (2003) 'The development of psychopathology from infancy to adulthood: The mysterious unfolding of disturbance in time.' *Infant Mental Health Journal 24*, 212–239.

Fonagy, P., Gergely, G. and Target, M. (2007) 'The parent–infant dyad and the construction of the subjective self.' *Journal of Child Psychology and Psychiatry 48*, 3, 4, 288–328.

Fonagy, P. and Target, M. (1997) 'Attachment and reflective function: Their role in self-organization.' *Development and Psychopathology 9*, 679–700.

Ford, T., Vostanis, P., Meltzer, H. and Goodman, R. (2007) 'Psychiatric disorder among British children looked after by local authorities: Comparison with children living in private households.' *The British Journal of Psychiatry 190*, 319–325.

Franklin, C., Kelly, M. S. and Kim, J. S. (2008) *Solution-Focused Brief Therapy in Schools: A 360-Degree View of Research and Practice.* London: Oxford Scholarship.

Friberg, J. (2010) 'Considerations for test selection: How do validity and reliability impact diagnostic decisions? *Child Language Teaching and Therapy 26*, 1, 77–92.

Fujiki, M., Brinton, B. and Clarke, D. (2002) 'Emotion regulation in children with specific language impairment.' *Language, Speech and Hearing Services in Schools 33*, 102–111.

Fujiki, M., Brinton, B., Isaacson, T. and Summers, C. (2001) 'Social behaviors of children with language impairment on the playground.' *Language, Speech and Hearing Services in Schools 32*, 101–113.

Fukkink, R. G. (2008) 'Video feedback in widescreen: A meta-analysis of family programs.' *Clinical Psychology Review 28*, 904–916.

Fukkink, R. G. and Tavecchio, L. W. C. (2007) 'Effects of video interaction analysis in a child care context.' *Pedagogische Studen 84*, 1, 55–70.

Fukkink, R. G. and Tavecchio, L. W. C. (2010) 'Effects of video interaction guidance on early childhood teachers.' *Teaching and Teacher Education 26*, 1652–1659.

Fulk, B. M., Brugham, F. J. and Lohman, D. A. (1998) 'Motivation and self-regulation. a comparison of students with learning and behavioural problems.' *Remedial and Special Education 19*, 5, 300–309.

Gallagher, T. M. (1999) 'Interrelationships among children's language, behaviour and emotional problems.' *Topics in Language Disorder 19*, 2, 1–15.

Gardner, H., Froud, K., McClelland, A. and van der Lely, H. K. (2006) 'Development of the Grammar and Phonology Screening (GAPS) test to assess key markers of specific language and literacy difficulties in young children.' *International Journal of Language and Communication Disorders 41*, 5, 513–40.

Gascoigne, M. (2006) *Supporting children with speech, language and communication needs within integrated children's services*, RCSLT Position Paper, RCSLT: London.

Geoffroy, M. C., Côté, S. M., Borge, A. I., Larouche, F., Séguin, J. R. and Rutter, M. (2007) 'Association between non-maternal care in the first year of life and children's receptive language skills prior to school entry: The moderating role of socio-economic status.' *Journal of Child Psychology and Psychiatry 48*, 490–497.

Gerhardt, S. (2004) *Why Love Matters: How Affection Shapes a Baby's Brain*. London: Routledge.

Gershenson, R. A., Lyon, A. R. and Budd, K. S. (2010) 'Promoting positive interactions in the classroom: Adapting parent–child interaction therapy as a universal prevention program.' *Education and Treatment of Children 33*, 3, 261–287.

Gesten, M., Coster, W., Schneider-Rosen, K., Carlson, V. and Ciccheti, D. (1986) 'The Socio-Economic Bases of Communication Functioning: Quality of Attachment, Language Development and Early Maltreatment.' In M. E. Lamb, A. L. Brown and B. Rogoff (eds) *Advances in Development Psychology 4*. Hillsdale, NJ: Erlbaum.

Giddan, J. J., Milling, L. and Campbell, N. B. (1996) 'Unrecognised Language and speech deficits in preadolescent psychiatric inpatients.' *American Journal of Orthopsychiatry 66*, 1, 291–295.

Gilligan, P. and Mamby, M. (2008) 'The common assessment framework: Does the reality match the rhetoric?' *Child and Family Social Work 13*, 2, 177–187.

Gilmour, J., Hill, B., Place, M. and Skuse, D. H. (2004) 'Social communication deficits in conduct disorder: A clinical and community survey.' *Journal of Child Psychology and Psychiatry 45*, 5, 967–978.

Ginsburg, K. R., The Committee on Communications and The Committee on Psychosocial Aspects of Child and Family Health (2007) 'The importance of play in promoting healthy child development and maintaining strong parent–child bonds.' *Pediatrics 1*, 119.

Girolametto, L., Weitzman, E. and Lieshout, R. (2000) 'Directiveness in teachers' language input to toddlers and preschoolers in daycare.' *Journal of Speech, Language and Hearing Research 43*, 1101–1114.

Girolametto, L., Weitzman, E. and Greenberg, J. (2005) 'Supporting peer interactions of children with low social communication skills.' *Journal of Speech-Language Pathology and Audiology 29*, 14–26.

Girolametto, L., Weitzman, E., Wiigs, M. and Pearce, P. S. (1999) 'The relationship between maternal language measures and language development in toddlers with expressive vocabulary delays.' *American Journal of Speech-Language Pathology 8*, 364–374.

Glass, N. (2001) 'What works for children: The political issues.' *Children and Society 15*, 14–20.

Glenberg, A. M., Webster, B. J., Mouilso, E., Havas, D. and Lindeman, L. M. (2009) 'Gender, emotion and the embodiment of language comprehension.' *Emotion Review 1*, 2, 151–161.

Gomez de la Cuesta, G. A. G., Humphrey, A. and Baron-Cohen, S. 'Evaluation of Lego Therapy.' Available at www.autismresearchcentre.com/research/project.asp?id=10, accessed on 22 January 2011.

Grady, C. L. and Keightley, M. L. (2002) 'Studies of altered social cognition in neuropsychiatric disorders using functional neuroimaging.' *Canadian Journal of Psychiatry 47*, 327–336.

Gray, C. (1994) *Comic Strip Conversations*. Arlington, TX: Future Horizons.

Green, J. (2006) 'The therapeutic alliance – a significant but neglected variable in child mental-health treatment studies.' *Journal of Child Psychology and Psychiatry 47*, 5, 412–435.

Greenberg, M. T., Kusche, C. A., Cook, E. T. and Quamma, J. P. (1995) 'Promoting emotional competence in school-aged children: The effects of the PATHS curriculum.' *Development and Psychopathology 7*, 117–136.

Griffiths, F. (2002) *Communication Counts*. Abingdon: David Fulton Publishers.

Gualtieri, C. T., Koriath, U., Van Bourgondien, M. and Saleeby, N. (1983) 'Language disorders in children referred for psychiatric services.' *Journal of the American Academy of Child Psychiatry 22*, 165–171.

Gureasko-Moore, S., Dupaul, G. I. and White, G. P. (2006) 'The effects of self-management in general education classrooms on the organizational skills of adolescents with ADHD.' *Behavior Modification 30*, 2, 159–183.

Hagaman, J. L., Trout, A. L., DeSalvo, C., Gehringer, R. and Epstein, M. H. (2010) 'The academic and functional academic skills of youth who are at risk for language impairment in residential care.' *Language, Speech and Hearing Services in Schools 41*, 14–22.

Hagberg, B. S., Miniscalco, C. and Gillberg, C. (2010) 'Clinic attenders with autism or attention-deficit/hyperactivity disorder: Cognitive profile at school age and its relationship to preschool indicators of language delay.' *Research in Developmental Disabilities 31*, 1–8.

Haight, W. and Sachs, K. (1995) 'The portrayal of negative emotions during mother–child pretend play.' *Child Development 69*, 33–46.

Hancock, T. B., Kaiser, A. P. and Delaney, E. M. (2002) 'Strategies to support language and positive behavior.' *Topics in Early Childhood Special Education 22*, 4, 191–212.

Hannus, S., Kauppila, T. and Launonen, K. (2009) 'Increasing prevalence of specific language impairment (SLI) in primary healthcare of a Finnish town, 1989–99.' *International Journal of Language and Communication Disorders 44*, 1, 79–97.

Hart, B. and Risley, T. (1995) *Meaningful Differences in the Everyday Experience of Young American Children*. Baltimore, MD: Brookes.

Hasson, N. and Botting, N. (2010) 'Dynamic assessment of children with language impairments: A pilot study.' *Child Language Teaching and Therapy 26*, 249–272.

Hayiou-Thomas, M. E. (2008) 'Genetic and environmental influences on early speech, language and literacy development.' *Journal of Communication Disorders 41*, 5, 397–408.

Haynes, C. and Naidoo, S. (1991) *Children with specific speech and language Impairment (Clinics in Developmental Medicine 119)*. Oxford: MacKeith Press/Blackwells Scientific.

Hazell, P. (2007) 'Does the treatment of mental disorders in childhood lead to a healthier adulthood?' *Current Opinion in Psychiatry 20*, 4, 315–318.

Heneker, S. (2005) 'Speech and language therapy support for pupils with behavioural, emotional and social difficulties (BESD) – a pilot project.' *British Journal of Special Education 32*, 2, 86.

Herrenkohl, T. I. and Herrenkohl, R. C. (2007) 'Examining the overlap and prediction of multiple forms of child maltreatment, stressors and socio-economic status: A longitudinal analysis of youth outcomes.' *Journal of Family Violence 22*, 7, 553–562.

Hetzel-Riggin, M. D., Brausch, A. M. and Montgomery, B. S. (2007) 'A meta-analytic investigation of therapy modality outcomes for sexually abused children and adolescents: An exploratory study. *Child Abuse and Neglect 31*, 2, 25–141.

Hirsh-Pacek, K. and Michnick Golinkoff, R. (2003) *Einstein Never Used Flash Cards: How our children really learn – and why they need to play more and memorize less*. New York: Rodale Books.

Hooper, S. J., Roberts, J. E., Zeisel, S. A. and Poe, M. (2003) 'Core language predictors of behavioral functioning in early elementary school children: Concurrent and longitudinal findings.' *Behavioral Disorders 29*, 1, 10–21.

Horton-Ikard, R. and Weismer, S. E. (2007) 'A preliminary examination of vocabulary and word learning in African-American toddlers from middle and low socio-economic status homes.' *American Journal of Speech-Language Pathology 16*, 381–392.

Huang, R-J., Hopkins, J. and Nippold, M. (1997) 'Satisfaction with standardized language testing: A survey of speech-language pathologists.' *Language Speech and Hearing Services in Schools 28*, 12–29.

Hughes, C., White, A., Sharpen, J. and Dunn, J. (2000) 'Antisocial, angry, and unsympathetic: "Hard to manage" preschoolers' peer problems and possible cognitive influences.' *Journal of Child Psychology and Psychiatry 41*, 2, 169–179.

Hughes, C., Jaffee, S. R., Happe, F., Taylor, A., Caspi, A. and Moffitt, T. E. (2005) 'Origins of individual differences in theory of mind: From nature to nurture?' *Child Development 76*, 2, 356–370.

Hughes, D. M., Turkstra, L. S. and Wulfeck, B. B. (2009) 'Parent and self-ratings of executive function in adolescents with specific language impairment.' International *Journal of Language and Communication Disorders 44*, 6, 901–91.

Huh, D. (2006) 'Does problem behaviour elicit poor parenting? A prospective study of adolescent girls.' *Journal of Adolescent Research 21*, 2, 185–204.

Humphrey, N., Lendrum, A. and Wigelsworth, M. (2010) *Social and Emotional Aspects of Learning (SEAL) Programme in Secondary Schools: National Evaluation.* Research Report. No. DFE-RR049.

Humphrey, N., Kalambouka, A., Bolton, J., Lendrum, A., Wigelsworth, M., Lennie, C. and Farrell, P. (2008) *Primary Social and Emotional Aspects of Learning (SEAL) Evaluation of Small Group Work.* Research Report. No. DCSF-RR064.

Hurwitz, S. C. (2002/2003) 'To be successful: Let them play!' *Child Education 79*, 101–102.

Huttenlocher, J., Vasilyeva, M., Waterfall, H. R., Vevea, J. L. and Hedges, L. V. (2007) 'The varieties of speech to young children.' *Developmental Psychology 43*, 1062–1083.

Im-Bolter, N. and Cohen, N. (2007) 'Language impairment and psychiatric comorbidities.' *Pediatric Clinics of North America 54*, 3, 525–542.

Irwin, J. R., Carter, A. S. and Briggs-Gowan, M. J. (2002) 'The social-emotional development of "late-talking" toddlers.' *Journal of the American Academy of Child and Adolescent Psychiatry 41*, 11, 1324–1332.

Jee, S. H., Szilagyi, M., Ovenshire, C., Norton, A. *et al.* (2010) 'Improved detection of developmental delays among young children in foster care.' *Pediatrics 125*, 2, 282–289.

Joffe, V. L. (2006) 'Enhancing Language and Communication in Language-Impaired Secondary School-Aged Children.' In J. Ginsborg and J. Clegg (eds) *Language and Social Disadvantage*, 207–216. London: Wiley Publishers.

Joffe, V., Cain, K. and Maric, N. (2007) 'Comprehension problems in children with specific language impairments: Does mental imagery training help?' *International Journal of Language and Communication Disorders 42*, 6, 648–664.

Johnson, B. (2008) 'Teacher–student relationships which promote resilience at school: A micro level analysis of students' views.' *British Journal of Guidance and Counselling, Special Edition 36*, 4, 385–398.

Johnson, C. J., Beitchman, J. H. and Brownlie, E. B. (2010) 'Twenty-year follow-up of children with and without speech-language impairments: Family, educational, occupational and quality of life outcomes.' *American Journal of Speech Language Pathology* 19, 1, 51–65.

Jones, J. and Chesson, R. (2000) 'Falling through the screen.' *Royal College of Speech and Language Therapist Bulletin* 579, July.

Jones, K., Daley, D., Hutchings, J., Bywater, T. and Eames, C. (2007) 'Efficacy of the Incredible Years Basic parent training programme as an early intervention for children with conduct problems and ADHD.' *Child: Care, Health and Development* 33, 6, 749–756.

Kaiser, A. P., Hancock, T. B., Cai, X., Foster, E. M. and Hester, P. P. (2000) 'Parent-reported behavioural problems and language delays in boys and girls enrolled in head start classrooms.' *Behavioural Disorders* 22, 117–130.

Kaler, S. R. and Kopp, C. (1990) 'Compliance and comprehension in very young toddlers.' *Child Development* 61, 1997–2003.

Kalyva, E. and Avramidis, E. (2005) 'Improving communication between children with autism and their peers through the "Circle of Friends": A small-scale intervention study.' *Journal of Applied Research in Intellectual Disabilities* 18, 253–261.

Kaplan, P. S., Dungan, J. K. and Zinser, M. C. (2004) 'Infants of chronically depressed mothers learn in response to male, but not female infant-directed speech. *Developmental Psychology* 40, 2, 140–148.

Kazdin, A. and Weisz, J. (eds) (2009) *Evidence-based Psychotherapies for Children and Adolescents.* New York: Guilford.

Kelly, A. (2003) *Talkabout Activities: Developing Social Communication Skills.* Milton Keynes, UK: Speechmark Publishing, Ltd.

Kennerly, H. (2009) *Overcoming Childhood Trauma: A Self-help Guide Using CBT Techniques.* London: Robinson.

Ketelaars, M. P., Cuperus, J., Jansonius, K. and Verhoeven, L. (2010) 'Pragmatic language impairment and associated behavioural problems.' *International Journal of Language and Communication Disorders* 45, 2, 204–14.

Kim, J. S. (2008) 'Examining the effectiveness of solution-focused brief therapy: A meta-analysis.' *Research on Social Work Practice* 18, 2, 107–116.

Knox, E. and Conti-Ramsden, G. (2007) 'Bullying in young people with a history of specific language impairment (SLI).' *Educational and Child Psychology* 24, 4, 130–141.

Kopp, C. B. (1989) 'Regulation of distress and negative emotions: A developmental view.' *Developmental Psychology* 25, 343–354.

Kotsopoulos, A. and Boodoosingh, L. (1987) 'Language and speech disorders in children attending a day psychiatric programme.' *British Journal of Disorders of Communication* 22, 227–236.

Kreppner, J. M., Rutter, M., Beckett, C., Castle, J. *et al.* (2007) 'Normality and impairment following profound early institutional deprivation: A longitudinal follow-up into early adolescence.' *Developmental Psychology* 43, 4, 931–946.

Kuhl, P. K., Conboy, P. T., Padden, D., Nelson, T. and Pruitt, J. (2005) 'Early speech perception and later language development: Implications for the "critical period."' *Language Learning and Development* 1, 3 and 4, 237–264.

Lahey, M. (1990) 'Who shall be called language disordered? Some reflections and one perspective.' *Journal of Speech and Hearing Disorders* 55, 612–620.

Laing, G. J., Law J., Levin A. and Logan, S. (2002) 'Evaluation of a structured test and a parent led method for screening for speech and language problems: Prospective population-based study.' *British Medical Journal 325*, 7373, 1152.

Laplante, D. P., Zelazo, P. R. and Kearsley, R. B. (1991) 'The effect of a short-term parent-implemented treatment programme on the production of expressive language.' *Society for Research in Child Development abstracts 8*, 336.

Lareau, A. (2003) *Unequal Childhoods: Class, Race and Family Life.* Berkeley, CA: University of California Press.

Lauth, G. W., Otte, A. T. and Heubeck, B. (2009) 'Effectiveness of a competence training programme for parents of socially disruptive children.' *Emotional and Behavioural Difficulties 14*, 2, 117–126.

Law, J. (2000) 'Treating children with speech and language impairments: Six hours of therapy is not enough.' *British Medical Journal 4*, 321, 7266, 908–909.

Law, J. (2005) 'The links between language and behaviour and the implications for interventions.' London: National Association of Professionals concerned with Language Impairment in Children (NAPLIC).

Law, J., Boyle, F., Harris, F., Harkness, A. and Nye, C. (2000) 'Prevalence and natural history of primary speech and language delay: Findings from a systematic review of the literature.' *International Journal of Language and communication Disorders 35*, 2, 165–189.

Law, J. and Conway, J. (1989) *Child abuse and neglect: The effect on communication development. A review of the literature.* London: The Association For All Speech-Impaired Children (AFASIC).

Law, J. and Elliott, L. (2009) 'The relationship between communication and behaviour in children: A case for public mental health?' *Journal of Public Mental Health 8*, 1.

Law, J. and Garrett, Z. (2004) 'Speech and language therapy: Its potential role in CAMHS.' *Child and Adolescent Mental Health 9*, 2, 50–55.

Law, J., Garrett, Z. and Nye, C. (2003) 'Speech and language therapy interventions for children with primary speech and language delay or disorder.' *Cochrane Database Syst Rev. 3*, CD004110.

Law, J., Lindsay, G., Peacey, N., Gascoigne, M. *et al.* (2000) *Provision for Children with Speech and Language Needs in England and Wales: Facilitating Communication between Education and Health Services.* London: DfEE.

Law, J. and Plunkett, C. (2009) *The interaction between behaviour and speech and language difficulties: Does intervention for one affect outcomes in the other?* Technical report. In: Research Evidence in Education Library. London: EPPI-Centre, Social Science Research Unit, Institute of Education, University of London.

Law, J., Rush, R., Parsons, S. and Schoon, I. (2009) 'Modelling developmental language difficulties from school entry into adulthood: Literacy, mental health and employment outcomes.' *Journal of Speech, Language and Hearing Research 52*, 1401–1416.

Law, J. and Sivyer, S. (2003) 'Promoting the communication skills of primary school children excluded from school or at risk of exclusion: An intervention study.' *Child Language Teaching and Therapy 19*, 1, 1–27.

Lawrence, D. (2006) *Enhancing Self-esteem in the Classroom.* London: Paul Chapman Publishing.

Lazar, R. T., Warr-Leeper, G. A., Nicholson, C. B. and Johnson, S. (1989) 'Elementary school teachers' use of multiple meaning expressions.' *Language, Speech and Hearing Services in Schools 20*, 420–429.

Lazar, S. W., Kerr, C. E., Wasserman, R. H. and Grat, J. R. (2005) 'Mediation experience is associated with increased cortical thickness.' *Neuroreport 16*, 17, 1893–1897.

Lee, E. C. and Rescorla, L. (2002) 'The use of psychological state terms by late talkers at age 3.' *Applied Psycholinguistics 23*, 623–641.

Legg, C., Penn, C., Temlett, J. and Sonnenberg, B. (2005) 'Language skills of adolescents with Tourette's Syndrome.' *Clinical Linguistics and Phonetics 19*, 1, 15–33.

Lemche, E., Klann-Delius, G., Koch, R. and Joraschky, P. (2004) 'Mentalizing language development in a longitudinal attachment sample: Implications for alexithymia.' *Psychotherapy and Psychosomatics 73*, 6.

Leslie, L. K., Gordon, J. N., Meneken, L., Premki, K,. Michelmore, K. L. and Ganger, W. (2005) 'The physical, developmental and mental health needs of young children in child welfare by initial placement type.' *Journal of Developmental Behavioral Pediatrics 26*, 3, 177–179.

Letts, C. and Hall, E. (2003) 'Exploring early years professionals' knowledge about speech and language and development and impairment.' *Child Language Teaching and Therapy 19*, 2, 204–229.

Levitas, R., Pantazis, C., Fahmy, E., Gordon, D., Lloyd, E. and Patsios, D. (2007) *The Multidimensional Analysis of Social Exclusion.* Bristol: University of Bristol.

Lieberman, M. D., Eisenberger, N. I., Crockett, M. J., Tom, S. J., Pfeifer. J. H. and Way, B. M. (2007) 'Putting feelings into words affect labeling disrupts amygdala activity in response to affective stimuli.' *Psychological Science 18*, 5, 421–428.

Lindgren, K. A., Folstein, S. E., Tomblin, J. B. and Tager-Flusberg, H. (2009) 'Language and reading abilities of children with autism spectrum disorders and specific language impairment and their first-degree relatives.' *Autism Research 2*, 1, 22–38.

Lindsay, G. (2007) 'Educational psychology and the effectiveness of inclusive education/mainstreaming.' *British Journal of Educational Psychology 77*, 1–24.

Lindsay, G., Desforges, M., Dockrell, J., Law, L., Peacey, N. and Beecham, J. (2008) *Effective and Efficient Use of Resources in Services for Children and Young People with Speech, Language and Communication Needs.* DCSF Research Report, RW053. London: DCSF.

Lindsay, G., Dockrell, J. and Strand, S. (2007) 'Longitudinal patterns of behaviour problems in children with specific speech and language difficulties: Child and contextual factors.' *British Journal of Educational Psychology 77*, 811–828.

Locke, A. and Ginsbourg, J. (2003) 'Spoken Language in the Early Years: The cognitive and linguistic development of three- to five-year-old children from socio-economically deprived backgrounds.' *Educational and Child Psychology 20*, 4, 68–79.

Locke, A., Ginsborg, J. and Peers, I. (2002) 'Development and disadvantage: Implications for early years.' *International Journal of Language and Communication Disorders 27*, 1.

Love, A. J. and Thompson, M. G. G. (1988) 'Language disorders and attention deficit disorders in young children referred for psychiatric services: Analysis of prevalence and a conceptual synthesis.' *Journal of Orthopsychiatry 58*, 811–816.

Lundervold, A. J., Heimann, M. and Manger, T. (2008) 'Behaviour: Emotional characteristics of primary-school children rated as having language problems.' *British Journal of Educational Psychology 78*, 4, 567–580.

Lutz, A., Dunne, J. D. and Davidson, R. J. (2007) 'Meditation and the Neuroscience of Consciousness.' In P. D. Zelazo, M. Moscovitch and E. Thompson (eds) *Cambridge Handbook of Consciousness.* Cambridge, MA: Cambridge University Press.

Mackie L. and Law, J. (2010) 'Pragmatic language and the child with emotional/behavioural difficulties (EBD): A pilot study exploring the interaction between behaviour and communication disability.' *International Journal of Language and Communication Disorders* 45, 4, 397–410.

MacKinnon-Lewis, C., Lamb. M. E., Arbuckle, B., Baradaran, L. P. and Volling, B. (1992) 'The relationship between biased maternal and filial attributions and the aggressiveness of their interactions.' *Development and Psychopathology 4*, 403–15.

Markus, J., Mundy, P., Morales, M., Delgado, C. E. F. and Yale, M. (2001) 'Individual differences in infant skills as predictors of child-caregiver joint attention and language.' *Social Development 9*, 302–315.

McCabe, A., Boccia, J., Bennett, M. B., Lyman, N. and Hagen, R. (2009–2010) 'Improving oral language and literacy skills in preschool children from disadvantaged backgrounds: Remembering, writing, reading (RWR) imagination.' *Cognition and Personality 29, 4*, 363–39.

McCartney, E., Ellis., E. and Boyle, J. (2009) 'The mainstream primary classroom as a language learning environment for children with severe and persistent language impairment implications of recent language intervention research.' *Journal of Research in Special Educational Needs 9*, 80–90.

McCauley, R. J. (1996) 'Familiar strangers: Criterion-referenced measures in communication disorders.' *Language, Speech, and Hearing Services in Schools 27*, 122–131.

McCauley, R. J. and Swisher, L. (1984) 'Psychometric review of language and articulation tests for preschool children.' *Journal of Speech and Hearing Disorders 49*, 34–42.

McDonough, K. M. (1989) 'Analysis of the expressive language characteristics of emotionally handicapped students in social interactions.' *Behavioural Disorders 14*, 127–139.

McGrath, L. M., Hutaff-Lee, C., Scott, A., Boada, R., Shriberg, L. D. and Pennington, B. F. (2008) 'Children with comorbid speech sound disorder and specific language impairment are at increased risk for attention-deficit/hyperactivity disorder.' *Journal of Abnormal Child Psychology 36, 2*, 151–63.

McHugh, B., Dawson, N., Scrafton, A. and Asen, A. (2010) 'Hearts on their sleeves: The use of systemic biofeedback in school settings.' *Journal of Family Therapy 32, 1*, 58–72.

Mecrow, C., Beckwith, J. and Klee, T. (2010) 'An exploratory trial of the effectiveness of an enhanced consultative approach to delivering speech and language intervention in school.' *International Journal of Language and Communication Disorders 43, 3*, 354–367.

Meins, E., Fernyhough, C., Fradley, E. and Tuckey, M. (2001) 'Rethinking maternal sensitivity: Mothers' comments on infants' mental processes predict security attachment at 12 months.' *Journal of Child Psychology and Psychiatry 42*, 637–48.

Meins, E., Fernyhough, C., Wainwright, R., Das Guptam, M., Fradley., E. and Tuckey, M. (2002) 'Maternal mind-mindedness and attachment security as predictors of theory of mind understanding.' *Child Development 73*, 1715–26.

Meltzer, H., Corbin, T., Gatward, R., Goodman, R. and Ford, T. (2003) *The Mental Health of Young People Looked After by Local Authorities in England.* London: The Stationery Office.

Mencken, H. L. (1917) 'The Divine Afflatus.' *New York Evening Mail.* 16 November 1917.

Meredith, L., Rowe, M. L. and Goldin-Meadow, S. (2009) 'Differences in early gesture explain SES disparities in child vocabulary size at school entry.' *Science 323*, 5916, 951–953.

Merrell, A. W. and Plante, E. (1997) 'Norm-referenced test interpretation in the diagnostic process.' *Language, Speech, and Hearing Services in Schools 28*, 50–58.

Miller, A. L., Kiely Gouley, K., Seifer, R., Zakriski, A. *et al.* (2005) 'Emotion knowledge skills in low-income elementary school children: Associations with social status and peer experiences.' *Social Development 14*, 4, 637–651.

Mills, D., Coffey-Corina, S. and Neville, H. (1994) 'Variability in Cerebral Organization During Primary Language Acquisition.' In G. Dawson and K. W. Fischer (eds) *Human Behavior and the Developing Brain*. New York: Guilford Press.

Mooney, M., Statham, J., Monck, E. and Chambers, H. (2009) *Promoting the Health of Looked After Children*. A Study to Inform Revision of the 2002 Guidance Research. Report no. DCSF-RR125. London: DCSF.

Mouridsen, S. E. and Hauschild, K. M. (2008) 'A longitudinal study of schizophrenia and affective spectrum disorders in individuals diagnosed with a developmental language disorder as children.' *Journal of Neural Transmission 115*, 11.

Mundy, P. and Neal, R. (2001) 'Neural Plasticity, Joint Attention and Autistic Developmental Pathology.' In L. M. Glidden (ed.) *International Review of Research in Mental Retardation 23*. New York: Academic Press.

Murray, A. D. and Yingling, J. L. (2000) 'Competence in language at 24 months: Relations with attachment security and home stimulation.' *Journal of Genetic Psychology 161*, 2, 133–140.

Music, G. (2011) *Nurturing Natures: Attachment and Children's Emotional, Sociocultural and Brain Development*. London: Psychology Press.

Myers, L. and Botting, L. (2008) 'Literacy in the mainstream inner-city school: Its relationship to spoken language.' *Child Language Teaching and Therapy 24*, 195–114.

Nagy, E. (2008) 'Innate intersubjectivity: Newborns' sensitivity to communication disturbance.' *Developmental Psychology 44*, 6, 1779–1784.

Nagy, E. and Molnar, P. (2004) 'Homo imitans or homo provocans? The phenomenon of neonatal initiation.' *Infant Behaviour and Development 27*, 57–63.

Nation, K., Clarke, P., Marshall, C. M. and Durand, M. (2004) 'Hidden language impairments in children: Parallels between poor reading comprehension and specific language impairment?' *Journal of Speech, Language and Hearing Research 47*, 199–211.

Nelson, J. R., Benner, G. J. and Cheney, D. (2005) 'An investigation of the language skills of students with emotional disturbance served in public school settings.' *Journal of Special Education 39*, 2, 97–105.

Newman, R. M. and McGregor, K. K. (2006) 'Teachers and laypersons discerning quality differences between narratives produced by children with or without SLI.' *Journal of Speech Language and Hearing Research 49*, 1022–1036.

Newman, T. and Blackburn, S. (2002) 'Interchange 78.' *Transitions in the Lives of Children and Young People: Resilience Factors*. Scottish Executive Education Department. Available at www.scotland.gov.uk/Publications/2002/10/15591/11950.

NICHD Early Child Care Research Network. (2003) 'Does amount of time spent in child care predict socio-emotional adjustment during the transition to kindergarten? *Child Development 74*, 976–1005.

Nind, M. and Weare, K. (2009) 'Evidence and outcomes of school-based programmes for promoting mental health in children and adolescents.' Paper presented at the European Conference of Educational Research, Vienna, Austria.

Nippold, M. A. (1998) *Later Language Development: The School-Age and Adolescent Years,* 2nd edn. Austin, TX: Pro-Ed.

Nippold, M. A. (2007) *Later Language Development: School-age Children, Adolescents and Young Adults.* Austin, TX: PRO-ED.

Nippold, M. A., Mansfield, T. C., Billow, J. L. and Tomblin, J. B. (2008) 'Expository discourse in adolescents with language impairments: Examining syntactic development.' *American Journal of Speech-language Pathology 17,* 4, 356–66.

Noll, J. G., Shenk, C. E., Yeh, M. T., Ji, J., Putnam, F. W. and Trickett, P. K. (2010) 'Receptive language and educational attainment for sexually abused females.' *Pediatrics 126,* 3, e615–e622.

Norbury, C. F. (2005) 'The relationship between theory of mind and metaphor: Evidence from children with language impairment and autistic spectrum disorder.' *British Journal of Developmental Psychology 23,* 3, 383–399.

Novick, R. (1998) 'The comfort corner: Fostering resiliency and emotional intelligence.' *Childhood Education 74,* 4, 200–204.

Nungesser, N. R. and Watkins, R. V. (2005). 'Preschool teachers' perceptions and reactions to challenging classroom behavior: Implications for speech-language pathologists.' *Language, Speech and Hearing Services in Schools 36,* 139–151.

O'Connor, T. G. and Scott, S. B. C. (2007) *Parenting and Outcomes for Children.* London: The Joseph Rowntree Foundation.

O'Neill, D. K. (2007) 'The language use inventory for young children: A parent-report measure of pragmatic language development for 18- to 47-month-old children.' *Journal of Speech, Language and Hearing Research 50,* 214–228.

Office for National Statistics (2005) *Mental Health of Children and Young People in Great Britain, 2004.* London: HMSO. Available at www.statistics.gov.uk/downloads/theme_health/summaryreport.pdf, accessed on 24 January 2011.

Ofsted (2006) 'Inclusion: Does it matter where pupils are taught?' Reference no. HMI 2535.

Ofsted (2008a) 'Looked after children – good practice in schools.' Reference no. 070172.

Ofsted (2008b) 'Good practice in re-engaging disaffected and reluctant students in secondary schools.' Reference no. 070255.

Ofsted (2009) 'The impact of integrated services on children and their families in Sure Start children's centres.' Reference no. 080253.

Ofsted (2010a) 'An evaluation of the provision of mental health services for looked after young people over the age of 16 accommodated in residential settings.' Reference no. 080260.

Ofsted (2010b) 'Transition through detention and custody: Arrangements for learning and skills for young people in custodial or secure settings.' Reference no. 090115.

Olds, D. L. (2006) 'The nurse–family partnership: An evidence based preventive intervention.' *Infant Mental Health Journal 27,* 1, 5–25.

Oliver, B. R. and Plomin, R. (2007) 'Twins' Early Development Study (TEDS): A multivariate, longitudinal genetic investigation of language, cognition and behavior problems from childhood through adolescence.' *Twin Research and Human Genetics 10,* 1, 96–105.

Ollsen, M. B and Hwang, C. P. (2001) 'Depression in mothers and fathers of children with intellectual disability.' *Journal of Intellectual Disability Research 45,* 535–43.

Ostrov, J. M. and Godleski, S. A. (2007) 'Relational aggression, victimisation and language development implications for practice.' *Topics in Language Disorders* 27, 2, 146–166.

Palikara, O., Lindsay, G., Cullen, M. A. and Dockrell, J. E . (2007) 'Working together? The practice of educational psychologists and speech and language therapists with children with specific speech and language difficulties.' *Educational and Child Psychology* 24, 4, 77.

Panksepp, J. (2008) 'Play, ADHD and the construction of the social brain: Should the first class each day be recess?' *American Journal of Play* 1, 55–79.

Papaeliou, C. Minadakis, G. and Cavouras, D. (2002) 'Acoustic patterns of infant vocalisations expressing emotions and communicative functions.' *Journal of Speech, Language and Hearing Research* 45, 2, 311–317.

Paradice, R., Bailey Wood, N., Davies, K. and Solomon, M. (2007) 'Developing successful collaborative working practices for children with speech and language difficulties: A pilot study.' *Child Language Teaching and Therapy* 23, 223–36.

Parow, B. (2009) 'Working with children with social, emotional and behavioural difficulties: A view from speech and language therapists.' *Emotional and Behavioural Difficulties* 14, 4, 301–314.

Parsons, S., Law, J. and Gascoigne, M. (2005) 'Teaching receptive vocabulary to children with specific language impairment: A curriculum-based approach.' *Child Language Teaching and Therapy* 21, 1, 39–5.

Parsons, S., Schoon, I., Rush, R. and Law, J. (2009) 'Long-term outcomes for children with early language problems: Beating the odds.' *Children and Society* 25, 3, 202–214.

Patnaik, B. and Babu, N. (2001) 'Relationship between children's acquisition of a theory of mind and their understanding of mental terms.' *Psycho-Lingua* 31, 1, 3–8.

Pellegrini, A. D. (2006). *Recess: Its Role in Development and Education.* Mahwah, NJ: Erlbaum.

Peña, E. D., Gillam, R. B., Malek, M., Ruiz-Felter, R. *et al.* (2006) 'Dynamic assessment of school-age children's narrative ability: An experimental investigation of classification accuracy.' *Journal of Speech, Language and Hearing Research* 49, 1037–1057.

Pennington, B. F. and Bishop, D. V. M. (2009) 'Relations among speech, language and reading disorders.' *Annual Review of Psychology* 60, 283–306.

Perry, B. (2004) *Maltreatment and the Developing Child: How Childhood Experiences Shapes Child and Culture.* Centre for Children and Families in the Justice System: Margaret McCain Lecture.

Perry, B. D., Pollard R. A., Blakley, T. L., Baker, W. L. and Vigilante, D. (1995) 'Childhood trauma, the neurobiology of adaptation and "use-dependent" development of the brain: How "states" become "traits."' *Infant Mental Health Journal* 16, 4, 271–291.

Peterson, C. and Roberts, C. (2003) 'Like mother, like daughter: Similarities in narrative style.' *Developmental Psychology* 39, 551–562.

Peterson, C. and Slaughter, V. (2003). 'Opening widows into the mind: Mothers' preference for mental state explanations and children's theory of mind.' *Cognitive Development* 18, 399–429.

Pickstone, C. (2003) 'A pilot study of paraprofessional screening of child language in community settings.' *Child Language Teaching and Therapy* 19, 1.

Pickstone, C. (2006) 'Participation in SureStart: Lessons from Language Screening.' In J. Clegg and J. Ginsbourg (eds) *Language and Social Disadvantage Theory into Practice.* Chichester: John Wiley and Sons.

Pollak, S. D., Cicchetti, D., Hornung, K. and Reed, A. (2000) 'Recognizing emotion in faces: Developmental effects of child abuse and neglect.' *Developmental Psychology 36*, 5, 679–88.

Pons, F., Lawson, J., Harris, P. L. and De Rosnay, M. (2003) 'Individual differences in children's emotion understanding: Effects of age and language.' *Scandinavian Journal of Psychology 44*, 4, 347–353.

Powell, S. and Tod, J. (2004) *A Systematic Review of How Theories Explain Learning Behaviour in School Contexts*. London: EPPI-Centre, Social Science Research Unit, Institute of Education.

Pressman, L. J., Pipp-Siegal, S., Yoshinaga, C., Kubicek, L. and Emde, R. N. (1999) 'A comparison of the links between emotional availability and language gain in young children with and without hearing loss.' *Volta Review 100*, 5, 251–277.

Prizant, B. M., Audet, L. R., Burke, G. M., Hummel, L. J., Maher, S. R. and Theadore, G. (1990) 'Communication disorders and emotional/behavioural disorders in children and adolescents.' *Journal of Speech and Hearing Disorders 55*, 179–192.

Propper, C. and Rigg, J. (2007) *Socio-Economic Status and Child Behaviour: Evidence from a Contemporary UK Cohort*. London: London School of Economics, Centre for Analysis of Social Exclusion.

Pyers, J. and Senghas, A. (2009). 'Language promotes false-belief understanding: Evidence from Nicaraguan sign language.' *Psychological Science 20*, 805–812.

Ramey, S. L. and Ramey, C. T. (1992) 'Early educational intervention with disadvantaged children: To what effect?' *Applied and Preventative Psychology 1*, 131–140.

Ramsbotham, Lord (2006) In *Hansard*, 27 October Col. 1447. Available at www.publications.parliament.uk/pa/ld199697/ldhansrd/pdvn/lds06/text/61027-0007.htm#06102742000250, accessed on 15 June 2011.

Reck, S. G., Landau, S. and Hund, A. M. (2010) 'Memory for object locations in boys with and without ADHD.' *Journal of Attention Disorders 13*, 5, 505–515.

Redmond, S. M. and Rice, M. L. (1998) 'The socio-emotional behaviours of children with SLI: Social adaptation or social deviance?' *Journal of Speech, Language and Hearing Research 41*, 688–700.

Reichow, B. and Volkmar, F. R. (2010) 'Social skills interventions for individuals with autism: Evaluation for evidence-based practices within a best evidence synthesis framework.' *Journal of Autism and Developmental Disorders 40*, 2, 149–166.

Reilly, S., Bavin, E. L., Bretherton, L. and Conway, L. (2009) 'The Early Language in Victoria Study (ELVS): A prospective, longitudinal study of communication skills and expressive vocabulary development at 8, 12 and 24 months.' *International Journal of Speech-Language Pathology 11*, 5, 344–357.

Reynolds, A. J., Temple, J. A., Ou, S. R., Robertson, D. L. *et al.* (2007) 'Effects of a school-based, early childhood intervention on adult health and well-being: A 19-year follow-up of low-income families.' *Archives Pediatric Adolescent Medicine 161*, 8, 730–739.

Rice, M. L. (1993) 'Don't Talk to Him He's Weird: A Social Consequences Account of Language and Social Interactions.' In A. P. Kaiser and D. B. Gray (eds) *Enhancing Children's Communication: Research Foundations for Intervention*. Baltimore, MD: Brookes Publishing.

Rice, M. L., Taylor, C. L. and Zubrick, S. R. (2008) 'Language outcomes of 7-year-old children with or without a history of late language emergence at 24 months.' *Journal of Speech, Language and Hearing Research 51*, 2, 394–407.

Rice, M. L., Tomblin, J. B., Hoffman, L., Richman, W. A. and Marquis J. (2004) 'Grammatical tense deficits in children with SLI and nonspecific language impairment: Relationships with nonverbal IQ over time.' *Journal of Speech, Language and Hearing Research 47*, 816–834.

Rice, M. L., Wilcox, K. and Hadley, P. (1992) 'The Role of Language and Social Skills.' In F. L. Parker *et al.* (eds) *The Social Use of Language: Research Foundations for Early Language Interventions.* Baltimore, MD: Paul Brookes.

Riggs, N. R., Greenberg, M. T., Kusché, C. A. and Pentz, M. A. (2006) 'The mediational role of neurocognition in the behavioral outcomes of a social-emotional prevention program in elementary school students: Effects of the PATHS curriculum.' *Prevention Science 7*, 1, 91–102.

Rinaldi, W. (1992) *The Social Use of Language Programme. Enhancing the Social Communication Skills of Children and Teenagers with Special Educational Needs.* London: NferNelson Publishing.

Rinaldi, W. (1996) 'The Inner Life of Youngsters with Specific Developmental Language Disorder.' In V. P. Varma (ed.) *The Inner Life of Children with Special needs.* London: Whurr Publishers.

Ringeisen, H., Casanueva, C., Urato, M. and Cross, T. (2008) 'Special health care needs among children in the child welfare system.' *Pediatrics 122*, e232–e241.

Ripley, K. and Barrett, J. (2008) *Supporting Speech, Language And Communication Needs: Working With Students Aged 11 to 19.* Thousand Oaks, CA: Sage Publications.

Ripley, K. and Yuill, N. (2005) 'Patterns of language impairment and behaviour in boys excluded from school.' *British Journal of Educational Psychology 75*, 1, 37–50.

Ritzman, M. and Sanger, D. (2007) 'Principles' opinions on the role of speech language pathologists serving students with communication disorders involved in violence.' *Language, Speech and Hearing Services in Schools 38*, 365–78.

Robb, L., Simpson, R., Forsyth, P. and Trevarthen, C. (2003) *Satisfying and Effective Teacher-Class Communication.* Presented to the Early Child Education Research Association Conference, Glasgow, September 2003.

Robinson, J. L. and Acevedo, M. C. (2001) 'Infant reactivity and reliance on mother during emotion challenges: Prediction of cognition and language skills in a low-Income sample.' *Child Development 72*, 2, 402–415.

Rock, E. E., Fessler, M. and Church, R. P. (1997) 'The concomitance of learning disabilities and emotional/behavioural disorders: A conceptual model.' *Journal of Learning Disabilities 30*, 3, 245–263.

Rogers, C. R. (1961) *On Becoming a Person.* Boston, MA: Houghton Mifflin.

Rogers-Adkinson, D. L. and Stuart, S. K. (2007) 'Collaborative services: Children experiencing neglect and the side effects of prenatal alcohol exposure.' *Language, Speech and Hearing Services in Schools 38*, 149–156.

Rogoff, B., Paradise, R., Arauz, R. M., Correa-Chávez, M. and Angelillo, C. (2003) 'First hand learning through intent participation.' *Annual Review of Psychology 54*, 175–203.

Rose, R., Howley, M., Fergusson, A. and Jament, J. (2009) 'Mental health and special educational needs: Exploring a complex relationship', *British Journal of Special Education 36*, 1, 3–8.

Roseberry-McKibbin, C. (2007) *Language Disorders in Children: A Multicultural and Case Perspective.* Boston, MA: Pearson Education.

Roth, A. and Fonagy, P. (2006) *What Works for Whom? A Critical Review of Treatments for Children and Adolescents*, 2nd edition. New York: Guilford Press.

Roulstone, S., Peters, T. J., Glowgowska, M. and Enderby, P. (2008) 'Predictors and outcomes of speech and language therapists' treatment decisions.' *International Journal of Speech-Language Pathology 10*, 3.

Roulstone, S., Owen, R. and French, L. (2005) 'Speech and language therapy and the Knowles Edge Standards Fund Project: An evaluation of the service provided to a cluster of primary schools.' *British Journal of Special Education 32*, 2, 78–85.

Rowe, M. L. and Goldin-Meadow, S. (2009) 'Differences in early gesture explain SES disparities in child vocabulary size at school entry.' *Science 13*, 323, 951–953.

Royal College of Psychiatrists (2004) 'Mental health and growing up: Factsheets for parents, carers and anyone who works with young people.' London: Royal College of Psychiatrists. Available at www.rcpsych.ac.uk/mentalhealthinfoforall/mentalhealthandgrowingup.aspx, accessed on 23 January 2011.

Royal College of Psychiatrists (2008) *Cognitive Behavioural Therapy (CBT)*. London: Royal College of Psychiatrists. Available at www.rcpsych.ac.uk/mentalhealthinfo/youngpeople/cbt.aspx, accessed on 23 January 2011.

Russell, C., Amod, Z. and Rosenthal, L. (2008) 'The effects of parent–child Mediated Learning Experience (MLE) interaction on young children's cognitive development.' *Perspectives in Education 26*, 4, 28–41.

Russell, R. L., Greenwald, S. and Shirk, S. R. (1991) 'Language change in child psychotherapy: A meta-analytical review.' *Journal of Clinical and Consulting Psychology 59*, 916–919.

Rutter, M., Beckett, C., Castle J., Colvert E. *et al.* (2007) 'Effects of profound early institutional deprivation: An overview of findings from a UK longitudinal study of Romanian adoptees.' *European Journal of Developmental Psychology 4*, 3, 3332–350.

Rutter, M. and Mawhood, L. (1991). 'The Long-Term Sequelae of Specific Development Disorders of Speech and Language.' In M. Rutter and P. Casaer (eds) *Biological Risk Factors in Childhood and Psychopathology*. Cambridge: Cambridge University Press.

Sabb, F. W., van Erp, T. G. M., Hard, M. E. and Dapretto, M. (2010) 'Language network dysfunction as a predictor of outcome in youth at clinical high risk for psychosis.' *Schizophrenia Research 23*, 3, 204–222.

Saltzman, K. M., Weems, C. F. and Carrion, V. G. (2006) 'IQ and post-traumatic stress symptoms in children exposed to interpersonal violence.' *Child Psychiatry and Human Development 36*, 3.

Sammons, P., Sylva, K., Melhuish, E., Siraj-Blatchford, I., Taggart, B. and Elliot, K. (2002) *Measuring the Impact of Pre-school on a Children's Cognitive Process over the Pre-school Period*. EPPE Technical Paper 8a. London: The Institute of Education.

Sanger, D., Moore-Brown, B. J., Montgomery, J., Rezac, C. and Keller, H. (2003) 'Female incarcerated adolescents with language problems talk about their own communication behaviors and learning.' *Journal of Communication Disorders 36*, 6, 465–486.

Sattler, J. M., Feldman, J. and Bonahan, A. L. (1985) 'Parental estimates of children's receptive vocabulary.' *Psychology in the Schools 22*, 303–307.

Saxton M., Backley, P. and Gallaway, C. (2005) 'Negative input for grammatical errors: Effects after a lag of 12 weeks.' *Journal of Child Language 32*, 3, 643–672.

Schneider, N. (2009) 'Social stories improve the on-task behaviour of children with language impairment (and BESD).' *Journal of Early Intervention 31*, 3, 250–264.

Schoon, I., Parsons, S., Rush, R. and Law, J. (2010) 'Childhood language skills and adult literacy: A twenty-nine year follow-up study.' *Pediatrics 125*, 459–466.

Schultheis, A. M. M. (2001) 'Language needs of preschoolers with behavior problems.' *Dissertation Abstracts International Section A: Humanities and Social Sciences 61*, 12–A, 4734.

Scott, S., Sylva, K., Doolan, M., Price, J., Jacobs, B., Crook, C. and Landau, S. (2010) 'Randomised controlled trial of parent groups for child antisocial behaviour targeting multiple risk factors: The SPOKES project.' *Journal of Child Psychology and Psychiatry 51*, 1, 48–57.

Seeff-Gabriel, B., Chiat, S. and Roy, P. (2008) *Early Repetition Battery*. London: Pearson Education.

Seidenberg, M. S. and Zevin, J. D. (2006) 'Connectionist Models in Developmental Cognitive Neuroscience: Critical Periods and the Paradox of Success.' In Y. Munakata and M. Johnson (eds) *Attention and Performance XXI: Processes of change in brain and cognitive development*. Oxford: Oxford University Press.

Seligman, M. P. (2006) *Learned Optimism: How to Change Your Mind and Your Life*. London: Vintage.

Sharma, N. (2007) *It Doesn't Happen Here: The Reality of Child Poverty in the UK.'* Essex: Barnardo's.

Sharp, C., Fonagy, P. and Goodyer, I. M. (2008) *Social Cognition and Developmental Psychopathology*. Oxford: Oxford University Press.

Sheehy, K., Rix, J., Collins, J., Hall, K., Nind, M. and Wearmouth, J. (2009) 'A systematic review of whole class, subject-based pedagogies with reported outcomes for the academic and social inclusion of pupils with special educational needs.' Research Evidence in Education Library. London: University of London, EPPI-Centre, Social Science Research Unit, Institute of Education.

Sigafoos, J. (2000) 'Communication development and aberrant behavior in children with developmental disabilities.' *Education and Training in Mental Retardation and Developmental Disabilities 35*, 2, 168–176.

Sinclair, A. (2007) '0–5: How Small Children Make a Big Difference.' *Provocation Series 3*, 1, The Work Foundation.

Singh, L., Morgan, J. L. and Best, C. T. (2002) 'Infants' listening preferences: Baby talk or happy talk?' *Infancy 3*, 365–394.

Skarakis, D. E., Campbell, W. and Dempsey, L. (2009) 'Identification of children with language impairment: Investigating the classification accuracy of the MacArthur-Bates Communicative Development Inventory-III (CDI-II).' *American Journal of Speech-Language Pathology 30*, 1058–0360.

Skovgaard, A. M., Olsen, E. M., Christiansen, E., Houmann, T., Landorph, S. L. and Jørgensen, T. (2008) 'Predictors (0–10 months) of psychopathology at age 1½ years: A general population study in The Copenhagen Child Cohort CCC 2000.' *Journal Child Psychology Psychiatry 49*, 5, 553–562.

Snow, C. E. (1972) 'Mothers' speech to children learning language.' *Child Development 43*, 2, 549–565.

Snow, P. C. and Powell, M. B. (2005) 'What's the story? An exploration of narrative language abilities in male juvenile offenders.' *Psychology, Crime and Law 11*, 3.

Snow, P. C. and Powell, M. B. (2008) 'Oral language competence, social skills and high-risk boys: What are juvenile offenders trying to tell us?' *Children and Society 22*, 1, 16–28.

Snowling, M. J. and Hulme, C. (2006) 'Language skills, learning to read and reading intervention.' *London Review of Education 4*, 1, 63–76.

Snowling, M. J., Bishop, D. V. M, Stothard, S. E., Chipchase, B. and Kaplan, C. (2006) 'Psychosocial outcomes at 15 years of children with a preschool history of speech-language impairment.' *Journal of Child Psychology and Psychiatry 47*, 8, 759–765.

Spaulding, T. J., Plante, E. and Farinella, K. A. (2006) 'Eligibility criteria for language impairment.' *Language, Speech and Hearing Services in Schools 37*, 61–72.

Spencer, S., Clegg, J. and Stackhouse, J. (2010) '"I don't come out with big words like other people": Interviewing adolescents as part of communication profiling.' *Child Language Teaching and Therapy 26*, 2, 144–162.

Spencer, N., Devereux, E., Wallace, A. and Sundrum, R. (2005) 'Disabling conditions and registration for child abuse and neglect: A population-based study. *Pediatrics 116*, 3, 609–613.

Stacey, K. (1995) 'Language as an exclusive or inclusive concept: Reaching beyond the verbal.' *Australian and New Zealand Journal of Family Therapy 16*, 3, 123–132.

Stanley, N. (2007) 'Young people's and carers' perspectives on the mental health needs of looked-after adolescents.' *Child and Family Social Work 2*, 3, 258–267.

Stansbury, K. and Zimmermann, L. K. (1999) 'Relations among child language skills, maternal socializations of emotion regulation, and child behavior problems.' *Child Psychiatry and Human Development 30*, 2, 121–142.

Steer, A. (2009) 'Review of Pupil Behaviour Interim Report 4: Review of Pupil Behaviour.' Available at www.teachernet.gov.uk/wholeschool/behaviour/steer, accessed on 24 January 2011.

Stein, A., Malmberg, L. E., Sylva, K., Barnes, J., Leach, P. and the FCCC team (2008) 'The influence of maternal depression, caregiving and socio-economic status in the post-natal year on children's language development.' *Child: Care, Health and Development 34*, 603–612.

Stevenson, J., McCann, D., Watkin, P., Worsfold, S. and Kennedy, C. (2010) 'The relationship between language development and behaviour problems in children with hearing loss.' *Journal of Child Psychology and Psychiatry 51*, 1, 77–83.

Stokes, S. F. and Klee, T. (2009) 'Factors that influence vocabulary development in two-year-old children.' *Journal of Child Psychology and Psychiatry 50*, 4, 498–505.

Stringer, H. (2006) 'Facilitating Narrative and Social Skills in Secondary School Students with Language and Behaviour Difficulties.' In J. Clegg and J. Ginsbourg (eds) *Language and Social Disadvantage Theory into Practice.* London: John Wiley and Sons.

Stringer, H. and Clegg, J. (2006) 'Language, Behaviour and Social Disadvantage.' In J. Clegg and J. Ginsbourg (eds) *Language and Social Disadvantage Theory into Practice.* London: John Wiley and Sons.

Stringer, H. and Lozano, S. (2007) 'Under-identification of speech and language impairment in children attending a special school for children with emotional and behavioural disorders.' *Educational and Child Psychology 24*, 4, 9–19.

Swinson, J. and Harrop, A. (2005) 'An examination of the effects of a short course aimed at enabling teachers in infant, junior and secondary schools to alter the verbal feedback given to their pupils.' *Educational Studies 31*, 2, 115–129.

Sylvestrea, A. and Mérettec, C. (2010) 'Language delay in severely neglected children: A cumulative or specific effect of risk factors?' *Child Abuse and Neglect 34*, 414–428.

Tager-Flusberg, H. (2006) 'Defining language phenotypes in autism.' *Clinical Neuroscience Research 6,* 3–4, 219–224.

The Communication Trust (2010) '*Hello* – frequently asked questions.' Available at www.thecommunicationtrust.org.uk/~/media/Communication%20Trust/Documents/Hello%20FAQs%20November%202010.ashx, accessed on 8 July 2011.

The Communication Trust (undated) *The Speech, Language and Communication Framework.* Available at www.thecommunicationtrust.org.uk/~/media/Communication%20Trust/Documents/SLCF%20%20%20Final%20Version.ashx, accessed on 6 July 2011.

The Nurture Group Network (undated) 'The six principles of nurture groups.' Available at www.nurturegroups.org/data/files/Who_we_areFurther_Info/The_six_principles_of_nurture_groups.pdf, accessed on 17 June 2011.

Thiessen, E. D., Hill, E. A. and Saffran, J. R. (2005) 'Infant-directed speech facilitates word segmentation.' *Infancy 7,* 49–67.

Thomas, R. and Zimmer-Gembeck, M. J. (2007) 'Behavioral outcomes of parent–child interaction therapy and triple P – Positive Parenting Program: A review and meta-analysis.' *Journal of Abnormal Child Psychology 35,* 3, 475–495.

Thompson, R. A. (1991) 'Emotional regulation and emotional development.' *Educational Psychology Review 3,* 4, 269–307.

Thorne, J. C. and Coggins, T. (2008) 'A diagnostically promising technique for tallying nominal reference errors in the narratives of school-aged children with Foetal Alcohol Spectrum Disorders (FASD).' *International Journal of Language and Communication Disorders 43,* 5, 570–594.

Tirosh, E. and Cohen, A. (1998) 'Language deficit with attention-deficit disorder: A prevalent comorbidity.' *Journal of Child Neurology 13,* 10, 493–497.

Tomblin, J. B. (2008) 'Validating Diagnostic Standards for Specific Language Impairment Using Adolescent Outcomes.' In C. Frazier Norbury, J. B. Tomblin and D. V. M. Bishop (eds) *Understanding Developmental Language Disorders, from Theory to Practice.* London: Psychology Press.

Tomblin, J. B., Hafeman, L. L. and O'Brien, M. (2003) 'Autism and autism risk in siblings of children with specific language impairment.' *International Journal of Language and Communication Disorders 38,* 3, 235–50.

Tomblin, J. B., Records, N., Buckwalter, P., Zhang, X., Smith, E. and O'Brien, M. (1997) 'Prevalence of specific language impairment in kindergarten children.' *Journal of Speech Language and Hearing Research 40,* 6, 12–45.

Tomblin, J. B., Records, N. and Zhang, X. (1996) 'A system for the diagnosis of specific language impairment in kindergarten children.' *Journal of Speech and Hearing Research 39,* 1284–1294.

Tomblin, J. B., Zhang, X., Buckwalter, P. and Catts, H. (2000) 'The association of reading disability, behavioural disorders and language impairments among second grade children.' *Journal of Child Psychology and Psychiatry 41,* 473–482.

Toppelberg, C. O. and Shapiro, T. (2000) 'Language disorders: A 10-year research update review.' *Journal of the American Academy of Child and Adolescent Psychiatry 39,* 143–152.

Topping, K. J. and Trickey, S. (2007) 'Collaborative philosophical enquiry for school children: Cognitive effects at 10–12 years.' *British Journal of Educational Psychology 77,* 2, 271–288.

Torr, J. (2004) 'Talking about picture books: The influence of maternal education on four-year-olds' talk with mothers and pre-school teachers.' *Journal of Early Childhood Literacy* 4, 2, 181–207.

Trevarthen, C. (2001) 'The Neurobiology of Early Communication: Intersubjective Regulations in Human Brain Development.' In F. A. Kalverboer and A. Gramsbergen (eds) *Handbook on Brain and Behavior in Human Development.* Dordrecht: Kluwer Academic.

Tronick, E. (2007) *The Neurobehavioural and Social Emotional Development of Infants and Children.* New York: Norton.

Trzesniewski, K. H., Donnellan, M. B., Moffitt, T. E., Robins, R. W., Poulton, R. and Caspi, A. (2006) 'Low self-esteem during adolescence predicts poor health, criminal behavior and limited economic prospects during adulthood.' *Developmental Psychology 42*, 2, 381–390.

Turley-Ames, K. J. and Whitfield, M. M. (2003) 'Strategy training and working memory task performance.' *Journal of Memory and Language 49*, 446–468.

Tzourio-Mazoyer, N., De Schonen, S., Crivello, F., Reutter, B., Aujard, Y. and Mazoyer, B. (2002) 'Neural correlates of woman face processing by 2-month-old infants.' *Neuroimage 15*, 2, 454–461.

US Department of Health and Human Services, Administration for Children and Families (2010) *Head Start Impact Study: Final Report.* Washington, DC: US Department of Health and Human Services.

van Balkom H., Verhoeven L., van Weerdenburg, M. and Stoep, J. (2010) 'Effects of parent-based video home training in children with developmental language delay.' *Child Language Teaching and Therapy 26*, 3, 221–237.

van Daal, J., Verhoeven, L. and van Balkom, H. (2007) 'Behaviour problems in children with language impairment.' *Journal of Child Psychology and Psychiatry 48*, 11, 1139–114.

Vance, M. (2009) *Performance on Language Assessments by Children's 4–5 Years in the UK.* Presented at RCSLT Scientific Conference, *Partners in Progress: Spreading the Word.*

Visser, J. and Dubsky, R. (2009) 'Peer attitudes to SEBD in a secondary mainstream school.' *Emotional and Behavioural Difficulties 14*, 4, 315–324.

Voci, S. A., Beitchman, J. H., Brownlie, E. B. and Wilson, B. (2006) 'Social anxiety in late adolescence: The importance of early childhood language impairment.' *Journal of Anxiety Disorders 20*, 7.

Vygotsky, L. S. (1962) *Thought and Language.* Cambridge MA: MIT Press.

Wadman, R., Durkin, K. and Conti-Ramsden., G. (2011) 'Social stress in young people with specific language impairment.' *Journal of Adolescence 34*, 421–431.

Waldfogel, J. (2010) *Britain's War on Poverty.* New York: Russell Sage Foundation.

Washbrook, E. (2010) *A cross-cohort comparison of childhood behaviour problems Summary of preliminary findings from a project for the Sutton Trust.* Available at www.suttontrust.com/research/a-cross-cohort-comparison-of-childhood-behaviour-problems/, accessed on 24 January 2011.

Way, I., Yelsma, P., Van Meter, A. M. and Black-Pon, C. (2007) 'Understanding alexithymia and language skills in children: Implications for assessment and intervention language.' *Speech and Hearing Services in Schools 38*, 128–139.

Weber, C., Hahne, A., Friedrich, M. and Friederici, A. D. (2005) 'Reduced stress pattern discrimination in five-month-olds as a marker of risk for later language impairment: Neurophysiological evidence.' *Cognitive Brain Research 25*, 180–187.

Werner, E. E. and Smith, R. S. (1992) *Overcoming the Odds: High-risk Children from Birth to Adulthood*. NewYork: Cornell.

Wetherby, A. and Prizant, B. (1992) 'Profiling Young Children's Communicative Competence.' In S. Warren and J. Reichle (eds) *Causes and Effects in Language Disorders and Interventions*. Baltimore, MD: Paul Brookes.

Wheelwright, G. O. and Baron-Cohen, S. (2007) *Mindreading DVD: Teaching Emotion-Recognition to People with Autism Spectrum Conditions*. London: Jessica Kingsley Publishers. Available at www.jkp.com/mindreading, accessed on 23 January, 2011.

White, C. (2006) *The Social Play Record: A Toolkit for Assessing and Developing Social Play from Infancy to Adolescence*. London: Jessica Kingsley Publishers.

Whitehouse, A. J., Durkin, K., Jaquet, E. and Zia'stas, K. (2009a) 'Friendship, loneliness and depression in adolescents with Asperger syndrome.' *Journal of Adolescence 2*, 309–22.

Whitehouse, A. J. O., Line E. A., Watt, H. J. and. Bishop, D. V. M. (2009b) 'Qualitative aspects of developmental language impairment relate to language and literacy outcome in adulthood.' *International Journal of Language and Communication Disorders 44*, 4, 489–510.

Whitwell, J. (2002) 'Therapeutic Child Care.' In K. J. White (ed.) NCVCCO *Annual Review Journal 3, Reframing Children's Services*. Available at www.johnwhitwell.co.uk/index.php/therapeutic-child-care, accessed on 16 June 2011.

Wiig, E. H. (1995) 'Assessment of adolescent language.' *Seminars in Speech and Language 16*, 1, 14–31.

Winsler, A., Fernyhough, C. and Montero, I. (eds) (2009) *Private Speech, Executive Functioning and the Development of Verbal Self-Regulation*. Cambridge, MA: Cambridge University Press.

Woolfson, L., Whaling, R., Stewart, A. and Monsen, J. (2003) 'An integrated framework to guide educational psychology practice.' *Educational Psychology in Practice 19*, 4.

World Health Organization (1996) *Multiaxial Classification of Child and Adolescent Psychiatric Disorders*. Cambridge: Cambridge University Press.

World Health Organization (2001) *The International Classification of Functioning, Disability and Health*. Available at www.who.int/classification/icf, accessed on 24 January 2011.

World Health Organization (2007) *International Classification of Diseases (ICD-10)*. Available at http://apps.who.int/classifications/apps/icd/icd10online, accessed on 5 July 2011.

Zadeh, Z. Y., Im-Bolter, N. and Cohen, N. J. (2007) 'Social cognition and externalizing psychopathology: An investigation of the mediating role of language.' *Journal of Abnormal Child Psychology 35*, 2.

Zeedyk, S. M. (ed.) (2008) *Promoting Social Interaction for Individuals with Communicative Impairments*. London: Jessica Kingsley Publishers.

Zeidner, M., Matthews, G. and Roberts, R. D. (2009) *What We Know about Emotional Intelligence. How It Affects Learning, Work, Relationships and Our Mental Health*. Cambridge, MA: MIT Press.

Zeman, J., Klimes-Dougan, B., Cassano, M. and Adrian, M. (2007) 'Measurement issues in emotion research with children and adolescents.' *Clinical Psychology: Science and Practice 4*, 377–401.

Subject Index

Author Index

Page numbers in *italics* refer to figures.

Lightning Source UK Ltd.
Milton Keynes UK
UKOW06f0927251116

288514UK00002B/110/P